Advance Praise for Simple Chinese Medicine . . .

"Dr. Aihan Kuhn has created a brilliant coverage of Traditional Chinese Medicine's role in modern society. Global society, as evidenced by the groaning economy, is in great flux. Americans and other industrial societies can simply no longer afford to ignore preventative health solutions, and continue to opt for the vastly more expensive 'crisis solutions' of surgery or a lifetime of drug dependency. Projections are that in coming years the US health costs alone will exceed $4 trillion annually.

The Chinese character for 'crisis' is made of two characters, 'danger' and 'opportunity'. The global economic crisis offers great danger if we do not re-think our journey toward our future. However, it can also offer great opportunity if we allow crisis to help us adopt a new way of seeing the world. [I recommend that] Dr. Kuhn's book, *Simple Chinese Medicine*, be read by [our nation's] Surgeon General and the Secretary of Education, as TCM should become part of health education and physical education for all students, taught in age appropriate ways, from kindergarten through university. Dr. Kuhn's book is an important part of, and can help accelerate, a revolution of ancient health tools which can help Western industrial nation's leaders educate themselves, their populations, and their government's ministers in ancient mind/body tools that could save their societies trillions of dollars year after year, while dramatically improving the quality of life for their people."

— ***Bill Douglas***, *is the Founder of World Tai Chi & Qigong Day (www.WorldTaiChiDay.org), and author of* The Complete Idiot's Guide to T'ai Chi & Qigong. *Bill presented in a Tai Chi and Qigong DVD now made available for free to Parkinson's disease patients throughout the United States through their physicians. He has consulted for the National Council on Aging's national Tai Chi project, and presented for the National Parkinson's Association's national conference. Bill is an honored faculty member of the American Qigong Association; recipient of the Extraordinary Service in the field of Qigong award from the National Qigong Association, Team Leadership Award from the National Tai Chi Chuan Association, the Media Excellence Award from the World Congress on Qigong, the Lou Gehrig Hero Award recipient for educating ALS professionals about Tai Chi and Qigong; and Bill is the 2009 Inductee to the Internal Arts Hall of Fame, presented by the American Society of Internal Arts.*

❀ ❀ ❀ ❀ ❀

"Dr. Kuhn is a medical doctor trained with western medicine and learned her Chinese medicine in medical school and subsequently in special Chinese medicine courses. This unique experience made her eyes focus on both sides of these [healing disciplines] and to try and combine them. Her new book *Simple Chinese Medicine* is an excellent source for people who are thinking about natural healing and alternative treatments for different diseases. From her book, we can learn not only the concept of Traditional Chinese Medicine, but also how to treat disease. It was said that Chinese medicine is a full philosophical system, which consider prevention medicine as very important as treating diseases. Some of the pr————— about eating the right food and maintaining optimal body weight.

You can find many ways in her book to keep you healthy and to treat various diseases. As a Chinese medicine enthusiast and a physician practicing medicine in the United States, I recommend you read her book and consider Chinese medicine as an alternative option for your health needs."

— *Jinxing Jiang*, *M.D. Attending Physician, John Stroger Hospital, Chicago IL*

❈ ❈ ❈ ❈ ❈

"As I read *Simple Chinese Medicine*, I got more and more interested in the development of TCM. Dr Kuhn has the advantage of understanding both China and the US. She takes a system that developed in ancient China and presents it so that we can understand that context and make helpful connections to our own culture. [Even] the recipes are easy enough for reluctant cooks, like me!"

— *Victoria Medaglia*, *student*

❈ ❈ ❈ ❈ ❈

"Dr. Kuhn's understanding of Eastern and Western medicine contribute to a complete view of human health and well-being. Her ability to explain how environmental conditions like diet, exercise, and stress affect the body's biology is easy to understand and enjoyable to read. There are many stories taken from her direct experiences, which serve to further illustrate and clarify some of the Eastern concepts that are less understood in the West. The in-depth focus on herbal medicine, acupuncture, and even less well-known Traditional Chinese Medicine techniques was fascinating, and it is clear that Dr. Kuhn is an expert in this field."

— *Jim Agnetta*, *Engineer*

Simple
CHINESE
MEDICINE

Simple CHINESE MEDICINE

A Beginner's Guide to Natural Healing & Well-Being

Dr. Aihan Kuhn
C.M.D. DIPL. OBT

YMAA Publication Center
Wolfeboro, N.H. USA

YMAA Publication Center
Main Office: PO Box 480
Wolfeboro, NH 03894
1-800-669-8892 • www.ymaa.com • info@ymaa.com

ISBN-13: 978-1-59439-124-8
ISBN-10: 1-59439-124-6

20200227

Cover design by Axie Breen
Edited by Susan Bullowa

Publisher's Cataloging in Publication

Kuhn, Aihan.

Simple Chinese medicine : a beginner's guide to natural healing &
well-being / Aihan Kuhn. -- 1st ed. -- Wolfeboro, NH : YMAA Publication Center, c2009.

p. ; cm.

ISBN: 978-1-59439-124-8 ; 1-59439-124-6
Includes bibliographical references and index.

1. Medicine, Chinese. 2. Holistic medicine. 3. Qi gong--Health aspects. 4. Tai chi--Health
aspects. 5. Mind and body. 6. Self-care, Health. I. Title. II. Title: Chinese medicine.

R601 .K846 2009   2009928166

610.951--dc22   0906

Warning: Readers are encouraged to be aware of all appropriate local and national laws relating to self-defense, reasonable force, and the use of weaponry, and act in accordance with all applicable laws at all times. Neither the authors nor the publisher assume any responsibility for the use or mis-use of information contained in this book.

Nothing in this document constitutes a legal opinion nor should any of its contents be treated as such. While the authors believe that everything herein is accurate, any questions regarding specific self-defense situations, legal liability, and/or interpretation of federal, state, or local laws should al-ways be addressed by an attorney at law.

When it comes to martial arts, self defense, and related topics, no text, no matter how well written, can substitute for professional, hands-on instruction. These materials should be used for academic study only.

Printed in USA.

Dedication

This book is dedicated to my wonderful husband, Gerry Kuhn who has given me tremendous help in many aspects in my life. Our love and friendship have been a big part of my healing career.

Romanization of Chinese Words

This book primarily uses the Pinyin romanization system of Chinese to English. Pinyin is standard in the People's Republic of China, and in several world organizations, including the United Nations. Pinyin, which was introduced in China in the 1950's, replaces the Wade-Giles and Yale systems. In some cases, the more popular spelling of a word may be used for clarity.

Some common conversions:

Pinyin	Also Spelled As	Pronunciation
Qi	Chi	chē
Qigong	Chi Kung	chē kǔng
Qin Na	Chin Na	chǐn nǎ
Jin	Jing	jǐn
Gongfu	Kung Fu	gŏng foo
Taijiquan	Tai Chi Chuan	tī jē chüén

For more information, please refer to *The People's Republic of China: Administrative Atlas, The Reform of the Chinese Written Language,* or a contemporary manual of style.

The author and publisher have taken the liberty of not italicizing words of foreign origin in this text. This decision was made to make the text easier to read. Please see the comprehensive glossary for definitions of Chinese words.

Table of Contents

Preface

Living in the U.S. for almost 20 years has made me realize that I had to take control of my own health and return to my roots in Traditional Chinese Medicine (TCM). Although I was trained in Western medicine in China, I grew to appreciate how Chinese medicine can complement other healing modalities.

Once I was in the U.S., I began to prepare my body and my mind, and travel the road to a healthy lifestyle, based mostly on the wisdom of Chinese medicine. Eating right, not only for weight control, but also for healthy living as well; using natural medicine for regular body tune-ups, and doing regular and appropriate exercises to keep mind and body in the best shape possible has helped me immensely. By taking responsibility for my own health, my new road to healthy living, I now see Western doctors for minor ailments or annual checkups far less often.

Ever since starting a clinic based on Chinese medicine, I began to see changes in my patients' lives such as better emotional stability, improved physical strength, fewer medical complaints, increased self-confidence, enhanced daily energy levels, better focus with less brain fog, as well as fewer aches and pains. TCM can alleviate many ailments and is just as valuable as Western medicine in many cases. The healing effects depend on the severity and the duration of the illness, the patient's cooperation, lifestyle, diet, exercise and mindset, as well as many other factors. It is very holistic. Generally speaking, the closer you are to natural healing and the more open and disciplined you are, the better the results you may expect. You have to trust your own healing ability; it will happen. I invite you to open your mind to TCM. It has been used for healing for over 4,000 years in the Orient. When your mind is open and you open the door to nature and TCM, you let the natural energy come in; this is the beginning of healing process. I hope this book will give you enough information to open the door to this wonderful ancient Chinese healing art and human energy science.

Dr. Aihan Kuhn,
C.M.D., DIPL., ABT.
Master, Tai Chi and Qi Gong
Director and Owner of Chinese Medicine for Health
President, Tai Chi and Qi Gong Healing Institute

Acknowledgements

Simple Chinese Medicine is my third book. It is not hard for me to explain my knowledge of Chinese medicine; but it is difficult for a person whose English is a second language to write a book in English. It took a great deal of time and effort to figure out how to say things right, how to put the language into the right order and make good sentences. In Chinese, we speak and write in the opposite order from English, so we say "English speaks opposite". On the other hand, an English speaker could say we speak in the opposite order. To finish this book, I needed much help. Therefore, I would like to take this opportunity to thank all the people who reviewed this book, made many corrections for me, and gave me great deal of encouragement.

First, I'd like to thank Jim Agnetta, a wonderful student of mine, who did the first editing and went through the most frustrating stage of dealing with my "Chinenglish." He is my good student, my good friend, and my "Tai Chi brother."

I'd like to thank Joyce Cerutti for some of the art work that made the book seem more alive.

I'd like to thank my dear friends Marie Murphy, Peggy Trundy, and Nancy Peters, who were a constant source of support and encouragement.

I also want to thank my editor Susan Bullowa, a very knowledgeable person with a thorough understanding of this kind of art. She put so much of her time and energy into editing this book as well as my previous book *Natural Healing with Qigong*; I am very grateful.

I also would like to thank everyone who read my first book, *Natural Healing with Qigong*, and gave me so much positive feedback. Their positive feedback encourages me to continue my writing about Chinese healing arts.

Finally, I would like to thank David Ripianzi, my publisher who helps me to spread the word about ancient healing art. By his efforts, more and more people will start to realize the importance of being healthy, happy, fulfilled, and well. My knowledge could not reach so many people without his help.

Aihan Kuhn
March, 2009

Part I

Natural Healing in Chinese Medicine

Chapter 1

Healing in Traditional Chinese Medicine

What is Traditional Chinese Medicine (TCM)?

What is Chinese medicine? Many people have asked me this question over the past 16 years while I have been describing and teaching this subject. Still, people do not know what Chinese medicine is and how it can help people with disease prevention, healing illnesses, improving immune functions, as well as improving the daily energy level in the body.

Traditional Chinese Medicine (TCM) is the oldest and most complete natural healing methodology that brings the body to optimum health, or balanced health. It derives from the Daoist practice based on the Yin-Yang theory and philosophy, and the Five Elements that were devised by the ancient Chinese people as a method of defining and explaining the nature of all phenomena. These theories and philosophies, which play a major role in the development of medical theory, represent the mainstay of physiology, pathology, diagnosis, and treatment.

Chinese medicine has been used for healing and disease prevention in China for many centuries and is still very popular due to its effectiveness. Chinese medicine works in the human energy channels we call meridians, to unblock the energy

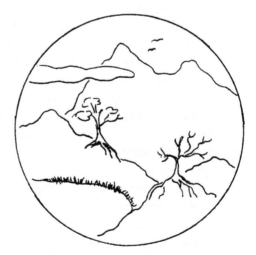

Chinese Medicine is from Nature

channel that goes through the whole body. Therefore, it treats the whole body rather than local symptoms. The methods that Chinese medicine uses (e.g., acupuncture, Chinese herbs, Chinese massage, a healthy diet and food healing, Chinese exercise, and a Daoist lifestyle) are completely natural without side effects. Chinese medicine uses multiple approaches involving mind and body healing and learning the natural way. This means that it will not work if you eat poorly and get no regular exercise.

When a person has optimum health, his internal ability remains strong and the adaptability of the body is superior. This is the key to health and longevity. When outside pathogens cause others to become ill, the person who has optimum health will not become ill. That is why in the flu season, some people get sick while others do not. In Chinese medicine, any excess or deficiency can cause body imbalance; the imbalance can cause the body to lose its ability to adapt to any kind of change, such as in the weather, food, drink, emotion, stress, and so on. Imbalance causes disharmony of organ energy that can vary in symptoms, which we call disease or illnesses. In Chinese medicine, it is called an energy blockage, poor blood circulation, or organ disharmony. The blockages in energy circulation consequently cause blockages of blood circulation; the blockages in the blood circulation can cause organ disharmony and, therefore many other ailments. In Western medicine, diseases are often attributed to a dysfunction of the immune system, abnormal levels of hormones and chemicals, and anatomical changes in the body that can be identified by scientific tests. Chinese medicine, on the other hand, sees the body from a different angle; it works in the human energy system rather than the structure of the body. We sometimes call Chinese medicine an energy medicine. Just like electricity, we can see the wire but not the flow of the electricity except when a spark comes from a short circuit. The goal of TCM is to create wholeness and harmony, restore the balance within a person, break any blockage in the body's energy channels, and promote energy and blood circulation. This not only initiates the natural healing process, but also speeds up the natural healing process. The results are similar to results of the Western approach—improved immune function, balanced body chemicals and hormones, and so on. Chinese medicine is a science, a very sophisticated science that requires a lifetime to explore. Having studied both Western and Eastern medicine, I believe that Chinese medicine is much more difficult to learn, more complex, and has more potential in human healing. TCM provides us with so much to explore.

Chinese medicine is a vast treasury of knowledge. It is the product of several millennia of practical experience in dealing with sickness. Chinese medicine can help relieve or heal all kinds of ailments with over 90 percent effectiveness treating non-traumatic ailments. It is a well-respected ancient healing art, a time-honored medicine that is now just beginning to be understood and recognized throughout the world for the tremendous benefits it can bring. Chinese medicine is practiced side by side and has equal value with Western medicine in China's hospitals, medical centers, and clinics. In China, people have the choice of both Western and Chinese medicine.

Not only does Chinese medicine have over 4,000 years of history, but Traditional Chinese Medicine also has its basis in well-defined theories and philosophy. Many areas in the world have their own medical traditions (e.g., Indian medicine, Native American medicine), but none is as grounded in theory and clinical practice. People from all over the world study Chinese medicine for healing and disease prevention. There are many TCM schools in China, and throughout the world, including the United States. More and more people have experienced Chinese medicine worldwide. There are more and more TCM practitioners each year. An increasing number of patients have improved health from this ancient healing art. The Western medical community has started to recognize this ancient healing method, and has begun to use acupuncture to treat patients in a number of medical facilities.

Natural Health—Creating a Healthy Garden

Health and gardening have very similar aspects. The human body is like a garden landscape. Appropriate sunlight, water, air, fertilizer, weeding, and monitoring of pests are important for plants to grow well and flourish. As they treat disease, Chinese doctors are like good gardeners. As in the garden, they enrich the soil by fertilizing the garden, balance the pH in the soil, eliminate bad insects, get rid of weeds, strengthen the roots of the plants, and improve the general condition of the garden. The garden will thrive through this maintenance program. Without this kind of attention, the garden will not be healthy. Think about an unhealthy tree: If you only spray chemicals on the leaves (thinking it will help), the tree might temporarily improve, but if its source is in the roots, the same problem will soon recur. If you improve and strengthen the condition of the roots, the tree will be stronger and grow healthier over a long time.

Human Self-Healing Ability

Every one of us is born with self-healing ability. When a person is injured with an open wound or you catch a cold, it is healed in several days or weeks, even without any intervention. Nevertheless, some people heal a lot quicker than others do, and others even get worse instead of better—the wound becomes infected or the cold turns into bronchitis or pneumonia. Even for cancer patients, some become healed, others remain in remission, and still others die. This has much to do with your healing ability, your interior landscape, your fundamental energy (Qi), and your organ system's "teamwork." Your healing ability is weak when your body's optimum health is lost; your organ energy is imbalanced; your fundamental substance of Jing (essence), Qi (energy), and Shen (spirit) is weakened; and your meridian system is blocked. Chinese medicine can strengthen your self-healing ability by improving your Qi and blood circulation in your body; strengthen the Jing; Qi, and Shen; balance organ energy; and unblock the meridian passages. All of this promotes your ability to heal quickly and fully.

Therapeutic Methods in TCM

As noted earlier, TCM is a methodology that involves many therapeutic methods. TCM modality includes acupuncture, Chinese herbal medicine, Chinese massage, and other related therapies (e.g., auricular acupressure, foot reflexology, magnetic therapy, and meridian therapy), Chinese exercise (e.g., Qigong, Taiji (Tai Chi) and other martial arts exercises), healthy diet, and using the Daoist philosophy to help deal with stresses of life. Daoist philosophy involves natural and harmonious ways of thinking, living, and dealing with life. Chinese medicine mostly works in combinations of multiple approaches. For instance, when you experience an acupuncture treatment, you also need to eat well and exercise appropriately. If you eat poorly, the therapy will not be as effective. These therapies or self-healing methods are used with the natural energies found within all living things that help the body heal itself.

Chinese medicine is used regularly by one-quarter of the world's population. In Asian countries, most of the population uses TCM. Its popularity has also been steadily increasing in the West as well as in the rest of the world.

What Chinese Medicine Offers

Health maintenance and disease prevention: Health maintenance is like a car or a house that requires periodic maintenance, but it is far important. Many people do not realize this. Therefore, when they have a health crisis, they are puzzled by it, they wonder why, and they are desperately looking for an answer. If they do periodic maintenance work, the crisis might be avoided. If we do appropriate maintenance work on our car, such as oil changes and tune-ups, it will last longer and be more reliable. If we take care of our house well, the house will remain in good condition for a long time. With good and regular health maintenance, you will not only have much less illness, but also have a good quality of life. What I call the "quality of life" is that you enjoy good health, good spirit, good mental attitude toward daily work and life. People think they do not need to exercise when they are healthy. Some children who eat poorly do not realize that it can affect their health when they become adults. People taking too much medication at a young age do not know the consequences of the long-term use of medication in later life. Young people who drink alcohol do not realize that it can affect their memory in later life. Overall, many things can be prevented if we do the appropriate maintenance and preventive work. People who suffer from heart disease, diabetes, cancer, lung disease, and other illnesses did not anticipate these problems earlier in their lives. They were healthy and they did not think that bad things could happen to them. The problem with some illnesses is that they are not reversible, so medicine can only relieve the symptoms. Chinese medicine is effective at preventing disease and Western medicine is effective in dealing with medical crises.

Healing illness: The effectiveness of healing in Chinese medicine has a long history. Chinese medicine has brought much happiness to peoples' lives by treating and preventing diseases ranging from injuries to tumors, from emotional disturbances to skin problems, from heart to kidney problems, from head to toe. Many therapeutic methods exist that help balance the body's energy and promote healing. Millions of people benefit from Chinese medicine. More and more people go to TCM practitioners because of the high efficiency of TCM care. People who experience TCM health care feel well. They obtain relief from their ailments, have more energy, and are more balanced. Some people obtain other benefits from treatments even though their original ailment may not improve due to prolonged illness, which has caused permanent damage. TCM practice has been shown to work very well in the human healing process.

Happiness and harmony in our lives: TCM can balance body energy, body chemicals, and hormones. If your body energy is balanced, your organ systems are maintained in harmony. You are unlikely to have physical problems; even if you were to have some physical ailments, they would be manageable. The balanced person is able to deal with stress and has a positive attitude and outlook. He would be less likely to overeat or overindulge himself, and less likely to have constant cravings for food and drink. He tends to stay calm and even-tempered. Even the upsetting feelings from a stressful event would be short and not interfere with daily life. TCM can relieve stress in a person by relaxing the tension in the body's energy paths. What I call quality life can help establish and maintain a happy and harmonious family and environment.

In 2002, I sponsored Duan Zhi Liang, a 97-year-old Qigong master, to give a Qigong workshop at my clinic. This old master was always joking, laughing, and singing. He was very mentally sharp and alert. He had such a good sense of humor that everyone who attended the workshop enjoyed him. He stayed in my house for several nights, but he slept very little despite having a full schedule of traveling and workshops. Obviously, he was in better shape than I was, because I was tired just from helping him in the workshop for several days. His Qi was so strong and powerful! I did not hear any complaints from him after a full day's work of seeing patients or giving workshops. Just imagine any 97-year-old seniors you have met—how many were like him? He is a perfect example for us all, because he has practiced TCM all his life.

Some people think that money can bring happiness. If money could bring happiness, then rich people would not have any problems, and they would have a perfect life. Unfortunately, this is not true. Money can only bring short-term happiness or temporary joy. Only living the balanced life can bring long-term happiness. In my practice, people who respect TCM and follow its philosophy recover more quickly than people who are inflexible, unable to change, and unwilling to do preventive work.

Longevity: Many studies in China have shown that people who practice Chinese natural healing in their lifetime not only were healthier but also lived longer. These studies focus especially on Chinese exercise called longevity exercise.

Differences in Chinese Medicine and Western Medicine

The Western medical approach is to treat the disease; the Chinese medical approach is to restore the body's energy balance and treat the whole person. Whereas Western medicine looks for abnormal test results, Chinese medicine looks for signs of disharmony and imbalance in the person. Western medicine will treat the symptoms by using medication, or remove the broken parts or extra growth with surgery. Chinese medicine harmonizes the person, strengthens the weak, gets rid of the excess, tonifies the depletion, dries the dampness, and promotes circulation of both energy and blood.

Western medicine relies on medical testing from technical support to evaluate test results; Chinese medicine evaluates the outcome and relies on the patient's overall feeling, the practitioner's skill in checking the tongue, pulse, and looking at the patient's spirit, and so on.

TCM practitioners pay close attention to the patient's lifestyle rather than concentrating only on the illness. They believe certain illnesses are caused from poor lifestyles and can be helped by correcting those lifestyles.

Because Chinese medicine focuses on health rather than disease, the best doctors in China are said to be those whose patients remain healthy. This is accomplished through supporting the body's natural balance, thereby enhancing the body's ability to defend itself against disease and maintain good health. We often make an appointment with a doctor when we are sick. We need them to tell us what is going on with our body, give us a diagnosis, and help us get rid of the pain and discomfort. Doctors are very happy if they can find a name for the problem, or can make a diagnosis. However, in Chinese medicine, the diagnosis is very different; it is not just the name of the illness. TCM refers to such illnesses as blockages, excesses or depletions, imbalances, Yin-Yang disharmony, etc. In addition, it advocates that we do not have to be sick before calling the doctor for an appointment. It is common to visit the

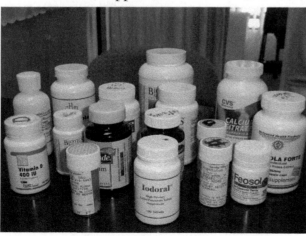

Western Medicines

TCM doctor for a tune-up treatment for minor ailments to prevent larger distress.

Take menopause, for example. Menopause is a group of symptoms caused by hormone imbalance. The body starts to lose estrogen; therefore, the amount of FSH (follicle-stimulating hormone) released into the bloodstream by the pituitary gland is elevated. Elevated FSH is the main cause of the symptoms. The Chinese medical explanation is that as we become older, our kidney energy starts to decline, causing other organ energy (e.g., liver, heart, spleen) to decline as well. These organs lose their coordinated functioning, or their teamwork, thus causing the various symptoms. The symptoms vary according to which organ energy is decreased or blocked. If a particular organ is weak, the patient will exhibit symptoms related to that organ. That is why one woman who experiences menopause could have different symptoms than others. In contrast, Western medicine treatment for menopause tends to supply estrogen to the body. This intervention permanently shuts down or dries up the ovaries. It is non-reversible. TCM treatment for menopause strengthens the organ energy and revitalizes the ovaries to enable them to continue releasing appropriate hormones until real aging starts. TCM treatments can restore the ovary function and delay aging. As can be seen, the two medicines provide different approaches. The disadvantage of taking estrogen is the potential for cancer in the future as well as speeding ovarian aging, whereas the TCM therapy offers no adverse effects.

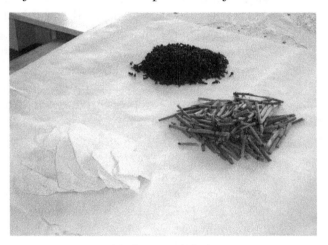

Medicine and Herb

Both medicines are important in our health care. Western and Eastern medicines are of equal quality and should be offered equally in our health care system to improve humanity's health and vitality. Both medicines are equally important and provide good results in treating various illnesses, so we should not say that one is better than the other is.

A Preventive Approach

There is an old Chinese saying: "You pay the doctor when you are healthy, you do not pay the doctor when you are ill" (but this certainly will not work in modern society). In the early years of China, when medicine was unavailable in most places, people's health was completely reliant on the "village doctor." The doctor's job was to keep people healthy. Patients paid the doctor to keep them healthy, not when they were sick. Our ancestors wisely stated:

> "The sages of antiquity did not treat those who were already sick, but those who were not sick...When a disease occurs and is only then treated, it's like waiting for thirst before digging a well, or waiting to go into battle before casting weapons"
>
> —*Huang Di Nei Jing*, known in English as *The Yellow Emperor's Classic of Internal Medicine*

These words were said by an ancient medical practitioner more than 2,000 years ago. They express the primary importance of preventive medicine. They are proof positive that Chinese medicine has long been valued as preventive medicine rather than emergency disease intervention. In China, the most difficult job for a doctor was serving as the Emperor's private physician. Centuries ago, the most prestigious doctor worked to take care of the Emperor. If the Emperor became sick, that doctor could end up being executed. It emphasizes the point that a high-quality doctor was judged by the health of his patients, not by how many sick patients he treated. That these preventive approaches existed for such a long time is due to the effectiveness of TCM in human healing and disease prevention. These natural methods improve the immune system, raise the energy level, balance body chemicals, and hormones, and delay the aging process.

As a result, for preventive work, Chinese medicine has more to offer than Western medicine, which is very good for emergency care and quicker relief of symptoms. Prevention and treating crisis are both important in health care. In some ways, the preventive work has deeper value than treating crises, even though treating a medical crisis may appear heroic. Preventive work requires more effort, which does not appeal to everyone. In my case, I would rather not have medical crises, which motivates me to do much more self-care and preventive work as possible on myself.

Treating Illness with TCM

Nowadays, Chinese medicine is used in treating various diseases as well as maintaining good health. Chinese medicine can treat the same diseases as Western medicine, (e.g., cardiovascular, pulmonary, gastrointestinal, endocrine, musculoskeletal, neurological, mental, genitourinary, sexually related, gynecological, immune system, autoimmune, dermatologic, or central nervous system disorders; addiction problems; infectious diseases; and much more. Oftentimes patients are surprised that TCM treatment helped to resolve their illnesses.

Western medicine can help relieve the symptoms of many illnesses (e.g., flu, or common cold, and many others) while the body heals itself providing comfort. The Western medical approach is to administer a flu shot to prevent flu, but there is no treatment for flu after a person gets it; there is only symptomatic relief. However, in Chinese medicine, there are many different herbal prescriptions for treating flu-types (wind cold or wind-heat). The symptoms of these two types of flu are dissimilar requiring different prescriptions. Even for the same type of flu, the prescription can vary for different patients.

To treat acquired food and other allergies, Western medicine gives antihistamines, or suggests a person avoid certain foods. TCM can eliminate the allergy most of the time. The outcome is that patients are able to enjoy most of the food they could not eat before.

Advantages of TCM for Treating Chronic Illnesses and Neurological Disorders

Chinese medicine is especially beneficial for chronic ailments for which Western medicine does not always cure, such as long-lasting muscle problems, arthritis, and pain.

All of these can benefit from acupuncture, Chinese herbs, and Chinese massage (called Tui Na, An Mo). Significant clinical evidence shows that acupuncture treatment for neurological disorders is very effective. A study from Harvard Medical School showed that brain sensory activity increased and nerve traffic to the brain was increased. In mainland China, people commonly have acupuncture treatments for neurological and muscular problems. In my practice, I have been able to help quite a number of shingles patients, who had severe pain. Within a short period, these patients were greatly improved after TCM care. Besides pain relief, most other symptoms were relieved, including skin rash, low energy, insomnia, and so on.

In many cases, both medicines treat problems with equally good results. For instance, Harvard Medical School conducted a study on depression, comparing acupuncture and Prozac. They found no difference in efficacy in treating certain types of depression, indicating that both acupuncture and Prozac can be used for treating depression. This study gives people hope that they can choose whichever medicine they like. In my Taiji school (The New England School of Tai Chi), two students have told me that they quit taking antidepressant drugs after practicing Taiji for a while. Even though this example only includes two students, it certainly indicates a possible value of Taiji for medical use.

For carpal tunnel syndrome, Western medicine uses surgery to correct the problem, but a TCM doctor uses acupuncture to restore the blood circulation to help the patient heal. Both Western and Eastern medicines are effective in treating carpal tunnel syndrome.

A 21-year-old patient had an ovarian cyst. Her doctor wanted to do surgery, which she feared. I treated her for three months with Chinese medicine and asked her to get another ultrasound afterward. By the end of the third month, the ultrasound showed no cyst and her symptoms disappeared. Therefore, both medicines can effectively treat ovarian cysts as well as numerous other cases.

Combining Chinese and Western Medicine

In some cases, either Western or Chinese medicine alone can treat illness with good results, but greater results may be obtained by combining these two medical systems. Having practiced as an obstetrician/gynecologist in China, I have seen many cases where the two systems, used jointly worked and provided excellent results in women's issues (e.g., infertility). For infertility caused by a structural blockage, Western medicine can help open the structural blockage to let the egg go through the tube; for infertility caused by a hormonal or functional problem, without the structural issue, Chinese medicine is the right choice. I have treated many cases of infertility with TCM methods, all with good results. These patients had no structural abnormalities but the infertility was caused by functional problems. Most people try Western medicine first, and then use Chinese medicine to increase the success rate. In fact, the combination of the two provides better results. There are numerous published articles in TCM journals documenting its effectiveness in treating infertility. In TCM hospitals in China, there are TCM gynecological specialists who only treat infertility with TCM methods. The benefits of TCM treatments for infertility include the regulation of female hormones to produce a large number of quality follicles; improved ovary quality to produce higher quality eggs; improved quality of the uterus, which provides a healthier environment for the egg; and strengthening the patient's Qi to help hold the embryo and decrease the chance of miscarriage. For patients who undergo in vitro fertilization, using TCM treatment can reduce the side effects from the drugs and increase the success rate.

Chinese medicine provides valuable natural health care and is just as important as Western medicine. They should be practiced side by side to provide quality health care. Neither medicine should criticize the other, no matter how effective it is. Every healing methodology has its own unique system, philosophy, and characteristics.

The Difference between Western Medicine and Eastern Medicine

Differences	Western medical science	Eastern medical science
Approach	Looking into structural problems, or chemical imbalances	Looking into energy problems, or organ disharmonies, blockages of energy paths
Correction strategy	Correct the body part where a person has a problem	Balance the body, correct the root of the problem
Diagnosis	Rely on technical support: X-ray, EKG, EMG, MRI, Blood tests, endoscope, etc.	Rely on the physician's experience and skills: tongue, skin, pulse, ear, smell, posture, diagnoses, etc.
Accuracy of diagnosis	More detailed, clear and easy to understand	Less detailed, vague and difficult to understand

Differences	Western medical science	Eastern medical science
Treatment	Can be invasive, high risk, side-effects of medication	Non invasive, very low risk, minimum side-effects
Medication distribution	Generalized drug	Individualized herbal prescription.
Results	Quicker, good in many cases	Slower, good in many cases
Self-/Preventive care	Less stressed	More stressed
Well received	Yes, internationally	Not yet, except in China
Treat Mind and Body	Less stressed	Very much stressed
For pediatric care	Good for emergency	Good choice for many cases
For urgent care	First choice	Not first choice
For chronic condition	Not good choice	Good choice
For injury	Not much to offer	Very good results
Hands on healing and psychological benefits	Not much	Yes
Cancer prevention therapy	Not much	Yes
Other	Structural or elements correction	Functional or energy correction

The Downside of Chinese Medicine

Even though there are myriad benefits from Chinese medicine, there are also some disadvantages, especially in the U.S. For example:

- No insurance coverage, which can be expensive for most people.
- For certain illnesses, long-term treatment is required before it is effective.
- Not effective in most urgent situations.
- In most cases, multiple visits are required.
- The taste of Chinese herbs is unpleasant and not tolerated by most people.
- Even though many people use TCM, the practice of Chinese medicine is still obscure.
- The diagnosis is vague, not easily understood by patients.
- The accuracy of diagnosis is not as good as Western medicine, which can clearly identify the problem from tests.
- Training of good practitioners is difficult, and takes a long time.

The Downside of Western Medicine

Western medicine is an excellent medical system that can relieve and treat disease effectively and quickly. It has readily available solutions for symptomatic relief that helps us function in our work and life. Medical technology gives us a very clear diagnosis that helps us understand how to treat the patient. The various surgical procedures are very important in certain ailments.

Still, there are some disadvantages to Western medicine:

- Side effects that cause other problems, some of which can be life threatening.
- Poor results for chronic illnesses, which make up most of the doctor visits.
- Risks of surgery.
- Less focus on preventive work.
- Difficulty in identifying and treating the functional problem, an area in which Chinese medicine does well.
- Focus of care in majority of cases is frequently on symptomatic relief.

Guidelines to TCM Care and Treatment

- Getting attention from Chinese medicine at earlier stages of an illness can result in much better results.
- For long-term and chronic illness, longer and more treatments are often necessary.
- Severe cases need more frequent treatments over longer periods of times than do minor cases.
- Younger people will get better results; children recover more quickly than adults do, and adults recover faster than seniors do.
- Medications (e.g., prednisone) can slow the healing process.
- Surgery can interfere with treatment if the incision cuts across meridians or important points.
- For faster healing, the patient's cooperation is important (e.g., diet, exercise, proper rest, restriction, follow treatment plan, and so on.).
- Functional problems are recovered from more quickly than structural problems.
- Patients with better mental and emotional health respond more quickly to TCM treatments.

Fifty/Fifty Health Theory

Many people do not see prevention and self-care as an important issue. They expect a doctor to fix them. Healing and self-healing require patience. Healing does not come the next day or next week. It relies on many factors. Everyone wants to be cured the easy way, taking the quick fix. We take far too much medication to achieve the quick fix, and then realize the quick fix does not happen every time. Healing involves a 50/50 effort on the part of both the practitioner and the patient. The practitioner or doctor takes 50 percent of the responsibility; he or she can help you restore the balance or the harmony and speed up the healing process. The patient should also take 50 percent of the responsibility by building a healthy mind and engaging in healthy activities that maintain the balanced, harmonious body energy. Exercise, diet, positive thinking, and a balanced lifestyle are all part of effective health maintenance. If you just rely on a practitioner without doing your part, your healing will only be 50 percent. You might improve temporarily but eventually your health will fall apart.

Taking Charge of Your Healing

A healthy mind plays an important role in the healing process. Everything you do comes from your mind. When your mind tells you to go to the doctor, you make an appointment. When your mind tells you to go for a walk, you open the door and go for a walk; when your mind tells you to avoid someone who is too negative, you do not call this person; when your mind tells you to make more money so you can buy a new house, you put in more shifts and work harder; when your mind tells you that you need to rest because your body is tired, you take a break or a nap, and so on. In human healing, once you develop a healthy mind, you know the right thing to do to make yourself feel better. You search for the answers and make the right choice, looking for the healing path (sometimes you make the wrong choice, but soon find out what you have done wrong and then you make it right). Your discipline will help you put in the effort to stay on a healthy path. You are then in charge of your own health. You know what is right and what is wrong. On the healing path, you should not look for results; this will cause anxiety that creates barriers for healing. When you are not looking anxiously for healing, healing begins.

On one occasion, a patient wanted to lose weight, and came to me for help. I told her that she needed to avoid eating late at night, which contributes to weight gain. I also pointed out certain foods that she needed to eat less of, but she told me that was not possible. In this example, she will have a difficult time losing weight. Treatment can help her balance her metabolism, but it will not help her lose weight if she eats too much fattening foods. During sleep, metabolism slows down; she cannot lose weight if she eats too close to bedtime. If she had taken this professional advice and had been willing to do her 50 percent, she might have been able to take off the weight.

History of Traditional Chinese Medicine

Due to the lack of evidence provided by historical records, we do not know the exact date Traditional Chinese Medicine started, but can only estimate the date from archeological findings. Over many centuries, the Chinese people learned to use anything from nature to enhance their quality of life. Besides learning about herbs and their uses, they learned which objects could be used to help heal. They also learned that weather could affect the human body. In the sixth century, acupuncture influenced Japan. In the seventh century, Korea started to teach Chinese medicine. Later, European and Arab countries started to learn Chinese medicine. In 1972, President Nixon visited China and watched a demonstration of acupuncture used for anesthesia during surgery and for other purposes. Ever since, the popularity of acupuncture has increased in the United States.

Early humans existed at least 125,000 years ago. There was no medicine. They died and lived entirely dependent on nature. Chinese medicine was first based on observations of nature and animals struggling to survive. Medicines were developed through observing the effects produced from using natural materials on different parts of the body, and seeing how an illness responded. Over time, people realized that nature held vast resources for medicine and healing. As they hunted for food, humans also found beneficial plants, stones, rocks, trees, dirt, shells, animal parts, minerals, and seeds to help heal injuries, alleviate pain, and reduce symptoms.

Early humans often became sick from eating raw meat, fish, and plants; they had many stomach, intestinal, and other digestive problems. When fire

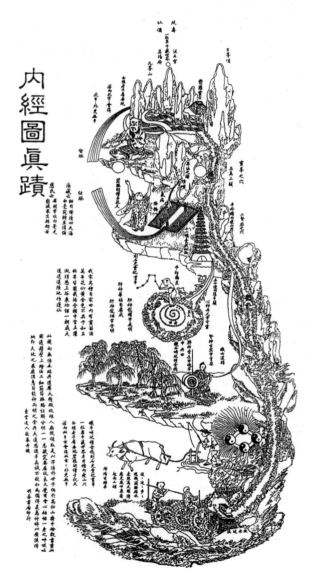

Classical Daoist illustration of universal forces at work.

was discovered, people started cooking the food they ate. They learned that gastrointestinal problems, as well as other illnesses, were significantly reduced. This was the first time the body was seen as a series of systems in which one organ can affect another. People gained the knowledge that stomach energy works better in warmth. The early Chinese also learned that certain foods and plants had the effect of decreasing pain and other ailments.

Heat Therapy: In the early years, the Chinese found that heat could reduce aches and pains caused by cold and damp climates. They used tree bark or animal skins wrapped around a heated stone, placing the stone on a wound or the painful area to decrease the pain. Later, they used burning herbs to relieve the pain and cold caused by illness. This was the origin of heat therapy and moxibustion. Cupping, massage, Gua Sha, and other therapies, which primarily treated the meridian system in the body, came later.

Acupuncture: Before metal was discovered, acupuncture evolved from the idea of using stones as instruments. In early days, people sharpened stones to make knife-edges that they used to cut open the infected skin to allow certain parts of the body to bleed.

The theory was that draining the toxic fluid would let the body heal itself. Some people became better at it while others died from bleeding (due to a lack of medical knowledge). In modern medicine, we adapt this technique to treat certain infections. The ancient Chinese discovered that when using this type of treatment for one part of the body, other parts of the body were also being relieved. This was the beginning of learning about the body's energy path, which we now call the meridian system. Later, sharp stones were made into the shape of a needle and inserted into certain parts of the body to reduce pain. Over time, the Chinese used objects such as animal bones and bamboo shaped and sharpened into needles; and even later, ceramic materials were used. As different metals became available, bronze, iron, silver, and gold were used for acupuncture. This was the beginning of modern acupuncture.

In 1968, in Chang Sha, Hunan Province in China, archeologists found an underground tomb from West Han dynasty (206 B.C.) containing an intact female body, along with nine acupuncture needles made from gold and silver. This discovery confirmed that our ancestors had used gold and silver needles to treat illness 4,000 years ago. Now, practitioners worldwide use stainless steel needles for treating an assortment of illnesses.

Today, too, acupuncture in China is mainly used for pain reduction and neuromuscular disease. Most Chinese use herbal medicine. Acupuncture is effective for treating all kinds of illnesses, not just for pain reduction. It is widely used in the United States; people undergo acupuncture treatments for many different reasons, from al myriad of illnesses to weight reduction, and even to delay facial aging.

Chinese Herbal Medicine: Chinese herbs were used even earlier than acupuncture, possibly as far back as 100,000 years ago. There were no written records that old, so no one can state positively when this practice began. Some of the earliest records that archaeologists found are characters referring to different herbs carved on turtle shell fossils. Herbal records were found only after there was a written language, beginning around 4,000 years ago. The Chinese discovered herbs by trying many different plants to identify the effects on certain discomforts. Some people died from the plants while others were healed. Some plants made the human body stronger while others made it weaker. Still others were beneficial when used in small quantities while others were toxic in large quantities. Certain herbs must be cooked in specific ways to be effective. Herbs include leaves, seeds, stems, roots, wild fruit, minerals, shells, and parts of animals. After years and years of practical usage of plants, the Chinese had collected a vast assortment of valuable information on herbs. The Chinese herbal medicine system is more complete then any other.

Chinese scientists and doctors who have done much research throughout all these years still continue their research to find more and more cures for illnesses, including cancer. In mainland China, most people use herbal medicine for different purposes. The popularity and use of herbal medicine is much higher than acupuncture and other therapies.

Publications in Early TCM History

The first complete herbal book titled *Shen Nong Ben Chao Jing*, which was written in the early Tang Dynasty (452-536 A.D.), listed over 365 medicinal herbs. That was right after Shen Nong had introduced agriculture to his people. The history, development, and use of this herbal book are well documented. The techniques described in *Shen Nong Ben Chao Jing* were very effective for treating patients for many years (e.g., Ma Huang for treating asthma).

The first medical book on TCM, *Huang Di Nei Jing*, known in English as *The Yellow Emperor's Classic of Internal Medicine* dates from about 200 B.C. It included information about the theory and philosophy of TCM as well as the benefits of acupuncture, herbs, diet, and exercise.

Materia Medica (Ben Cao Gang Mu) was written by Dr. Li Shi Zhen during the Ming Dynasty (1368-1644). He traveled all over China in search of medical herbs and spent 27 years describing about 2,000 different herbs. He searched mountains and rivers, looking for leaves, roots, plants, and trees; he dissected animals to identify their potential use. This book is an encyclopedia of Chinese herbal medicine that has information about almost 2,000 different kinds of herbal medicines. It is a very important TCM herbal reference book used by practitioners all over the world. This book added to TCM herbalist knowledge with the inclusion of more than 1,500 herbs discovered after those described in *Shen Nong Ben Cao Jing*.

There are many important historical publications about TCM, some originating from ancient sources, others were destroyed during wars, and still others were lost due to events such as the Chinese Cultural Revolution (1966-1976).

Doctors in Early TCM History

A number of excellent Chinese doctors have been dedicated to the discovery and development of Chinese medicine.

Zhang Zhong Jin (150-219) was a famous Chinese doctor who has the reputation of foreseeing illness. He wrote *Treatise on Diseases Caused by Cold Factors (Shang Han Lun)*, a useful guide to the treatment of internal disease that is still used today.

In the first book of internal medicine in TCM history, Dr. Zhang attributed disease to two evils — internal and external. The first volume describes external evils; the second volume describes internal evils; these two volumes covered the entire knowledge of Chinese medicine up to that time. Dr. Zhang was able to predict disease by looking at signs during early stages of illnesses. In one TCM legend, Dr. Zhang saw a 20-year-old writer named Wang Zong Xuan and told him that he had a serious disease; his eyebrows would fall off by the age of 40. The doctor suggested that he take an herbal medicine to prevent it from happening. Dr. Zhang gave a prescription to this young man. Wang did not believe him and did not take the medicine the doctor had prescribed; he thought Dr. Zhang was a fool. Sometime later, doctor Zhang saw him again and asked him if he took the herb that Zhang prescribed; he lied to the doctor saying that he took the herb. Dr. Zhang knew he was lying just by looking at him and asked him why he did not cherish his life. The writer still did not believe Dr. Zhang. At age 40, this young man's eyebrows fell off and he died six months later. The historian thought that Wang Zong Xuan might have been suffering from Ma Feng (a serious infectious disease from a virus that can stay in the body many years). This story indicates that our Chinese ancestors were able to identify the early stages of serious disease. Dr. Zhang wrote fifty-seven books about Chinese medicine.

Another well-known Chinese doctor named Hua Tuo, (145-203) had expertise in many specialties in internal medicine, surgery, gynecology, acupuncture, ear/nose/throat medicine, and preventive medicine (like Qigong exercises and Five Animal Qigong), which is still practiced by many Chinese in mainland China. He was the first Chinese doctor to use anesthesia for abdominal surgery. He was an excellent surgeon and TCM practitioner. During the Three Kingdom Period, an emperor named Chao Chao suffered from migraine headaches and asked Hua Tuo to treat him. Hua Tuo used one acupuncture needle that relieved Chao Chao's migraine immediately. Chao Chao wanted Hua Tuo to work and live in the palace (he was afraid of another migraine), but Hua Tuo refused to do so; he preferred to use his skills to help patients other than just the Emperor himself. Chao Chao was furious; which caused the headache to return. Chao Chao asked Hua Tuo to treat him again. Hua Tuo suggested that in order to get rid of the headache completely, he needed surgery. Thinking that Hua wanted to murder him, Chao Chao put Hua Tuo in jail. In the prison ward, Hua Tuo knew that his life would be over soon, so he asked the guards if they could help him save the medical documents and records containing his knowledge of TCM so they could be used to teach other doctors. These guards feared Chao Chao and did not dare to save Hua Tuo's notes, and they burned them, which is why Hua Tuo left no publications behind. Almost every Chinese knows his name and of his interest in preventive medicine.

Sun Si-Miao (581-683) who studied Chinese medicine from an early age was motivated by his poor health. He had such a wide range of knowledge that even the emperors of the Tang Dynasty (Tang Tai Zong and Tang Gao Zong) wanted him to work in the palace. He refused to do so and continued to work for all people. Of good moral character, he believed that "health is more important than gold." His *Golden Principle – A Guide for Medical Workers* stated:

> "When people come to you with a serious disease and ask for help, you cannot concern yourself with weather they are esteemed or dishonorable, wealthy or poor, elderly or young, beautiful or ugly. Your care must be safe and not swayed by whether you are a dearest family member or an adversary, your good friend or a stranger, Chinese or foreigner, foolish or wise. In your mind's eye, each patient is on the same level, degree, and class, and is treated as close as family. Your care must never be self-serving or motivated by what brings good or bad fortune, or by that which is pleasing or upsetting. Your protection and care should be precisely what is necessary: no more, no less, without deference to your own safety and life. Know, in your heart, that your good deeds are sincere and not a game. Show courage but caution. Actively implore and broaden your knowledge, but stand firmly on the principles of which you are certain."

Chinese medicine struggled to combat superstition, witchcraft, and lay people who used the name of Chinese medicine to perform foolish and deceptive procedures. It has overcome many obstacles and problems since the early years. After thousands of years, credibility and respect came to Chinese medicine because of scientific evidence, clinical proof, and improved human education and knowledge. Chinese scientists and doctors continue to research on herbs, medicines, and diseases. Every year, they discover more and more benefits from their research into herbal medicine, acupuncture, and Chinese massage, finding techniques that range from treating psoriasis to cancer, diabetes to heart disease, and muscle disease to mental illness.

TCM Medical Schools and TCM Doctors

Medical schools in China require students to study for five years. After graduating, there is a three-year clinical training program for graduates (similar to being a resident in the U.S.). Young doctors who have just graduated from school must work very hard before becoming comfortable with patients. It takes a long time to become a good TCM doctor. Since TCM is quite complicated, doctors must continue learning throughout their entire practice, their entire lifetime. Only a devoted doctor can become a high-quality doctor, one who would put a lifetime of effort into studying this kind of healing system. That is why in the Chinese tradition; many people prefer to see older doctors. They believe the older the better, which makes it difficult for young TCM doctors. There are young doctors who are devoted to TCM study and practice, and they try their best to make people feel better. As in any kind of work, experience is always an indication of skill, especially in medicine. From my own experience as a young doctor, over 25 years ago, I would advise a young practitioner to always be modest, and never think that you have learned enough. Anything that the practitioner encounters can be a new learning experience, even something unpleasant. Learning and growing by practicing TCM should never stop if you are dedicated to practicing Chinese medicine.

An interesting aspect of Chinese medicine is that the more you learn and the more interested you become, the more you will want to learn. It is a mysterious science where you can enjoy new surprises all the time. Some Chinese doctors only focus on treating illness while others focus on whole body and mind healing. The doctors who focus on the latter tend to have good discipline. If the practitioner practices what he preaches, it is much easier for him to educate and treat his patients.

An old Chinese saying—"If one practices medicine superficially, one should not practice medicine at all."—clearly states that doctors should be devoted to giving the highest quality care to their patients. In China's earlier years, people who studied medicine were not motivated by money; treating patients was all about the achievement and the satisfaction from being able to help people, and earning the reputation of being an excellent doctor.

Chinese medicine offers a huge potential in the healing process. There is another old saying, "Patients do not die from disease; they die from medicine." Every disease has its cause and its cure, except when we do not know enough to find a cure. Only dedicated and devoted doctors work hard to find an answer, a cure. They find answers for many ailments, but still need to explore in order to find more cures for disease.

TCM Theory and Sources

Traditional Chinese Medicine during its long existence remains popular today due to its effectiveness in treating and preventing illness.

Yin-Yang Philosophy

The theory that stands behind TCM is Yin-Yang, the principle of nature, or the way of nature.

The concept of Yin-Yang originated in ancient China as a method of defining and explaining the nature of all phenomena. Ancient Chinese present the concept of nature as being fundamental to all natural sciences. Not only medicine, but also astronomy, calendar science, geography, and agriculture made extensive use of and were strongly influenced by these theories. The Yin-Yang theory, along with Five Elements (which is described later), have played a major role in the development of medical theory and represent the mainstay of philosophy, pathology, diagnosis, and treatment.

The theory of Yin-Yang, derived from age-old observations of nature, describes the way phenomena naturally groups in pairs of opposites: heaven and earth, sun and moon, night and day, winter and summer, male and female, black and white, up and down, inside and outside, movement and stillness. You can also consider Western medicine as Yang and Traditional Chinese Medicine as Yin. The Yang is considered active, bright, upbeat, high key, moving; the Yin is considered passive, dark, down beat, low key, still. Yin and Yang aspects depend on each other. They balance each other and counterbalance each other. Without Yang, there would be no Yin; without Yin, there would be no Yang. Just as if there were no woman, there would be no man; without black to compare, there would be no white. Similarly, in nature, if there is not any bad, we will not know what good is.

Table Yin-Yang Categorization of General Phenomena

Phenomenon	Yang	Yin
Elevation	Up	Down
Sex	Male	Female
Sound	Loud	Quiet
Space	Heaven	Earth
Season	Summer	Winter
Color	White	Black
Time	Day	Night
Temperature	Hot	Cold
Weather	Sunny	Rainy
Weight	Heavy	Light
Motion	Fast	Slow
Food taste	Spicy, strong	Light, mild
Mood	Anxious	Depressed
Personality	High key, type A	Low key, type B
Body part I	External	Internal
Body part II	Upper body	Lower body
Organ	Hollow organ (Bladder)	Solid organ (Kidney)

These pairs of opposites are also complimentary in that they depend upon and counterbalance each other. Furthermore, they are mutually convertible, since either may change into its complement. The day eventually becomes night, the night eventually becomes day, the bad can eventually become good, and the good can become bad, too. In human life, we have healthy days and sick days, and the sick days eventually become healthy days. We have pleasant periods and unpleasant periods: The unpleasant days pass in time. This also teaches us that things do change; the "change" can go either way: positive or negative. When we are young, we are full of Yang energy. We are active, able to work long hours, able to tolerate hard physical work, and are able to do heavy work. However, our mind is still developing and immature, and we often make mistakes. As we grow older, our Yang energy diminishes and our Yin energy increases. We become less active, unable to work for long hours like we did before, unable to do heavy work; but our mind is much more mature, more clear and stable. We are wiser and we make fewer mistakes. Everyone has two sides: a strong side and a weak side (Yin side and Yang side), which makes everyone unique in their own way. We cannot say which is good and which is bad. All we need to do is adjust ourselves to be more accepting and open to the opposite. If you want to be a perfect person, or look for a perfect person to be your partner, or try to have perfect health, you might have problems, because it is not possible. There is no such thing as a perfect person, perfect health, perfect life, perfect husband, perfect wife, perfect job, perfect parents, perfect children, and so on.

Yin and Yang are rooted in each other, they are indispensable to each other, and are also mutually engendering. They are interdependent. As noted earlier, without Yin, there would be no Yang. Yin and Yang counterbalance each other. Extreme Yin can cause weakness to Yang, and excess Yang can cause weakness to Yin. In the human body, if you have an excess in one organ, another organ might be weak. In the human brain, if you overdevelop one side of your brain, the other side might be weak. That is part of the reason there are many artists suffering from depression. In normal daily life, if you focus on one aspect and ignore the other, you lose balance and might have other problems. Some people have great academic skill, but lack in social skills; they tend to have problems in their lives. Some athletes focus on physical development, but lack mental and spiritual development; they tend to have different problems in their lives. In business, you have a good year and a bad year, and you have gains and losses. You gain in some ways and lose in other ways. If you only want to gain and cannot handle the loss, you cannot have a good business because you do not understand the universal law—the law of nature, the Yin and the Yang. People who do not understand loss cannot gain. Yin-Yang is in everyday life; it is at the core of the idea of balance.

All occupations can benefit from understanding Yin and Yang concepts and Daoist philosophy (which is described elsewhere in this book). If a doctor is too busy and schedules too many appointments with patients, the quality of care that he can provide his patients will diminish. If a teacher has too many students, then the quality of the instruction he provides will also lessen. If we work 16 hours a day, we definitely need a good sleep, or we might lose our health. If we eat too much all the time, we will not only gain weight, but will also lose our health and energy. If we think too much, our mind will deviate or lose focus. In general, any excess or deficiency will cause some kind of setback.

The concept of Yin and Yang is not strictly black and white. When you look at the symbol of Yin-Yang, you will see a black dot inside the white part of the symbol, and a white dot inside the black part of the symbol. This suggests there is no absolutely right or wrong: If you think something is right, it might not be right to others; and if you think something is wrong, it might be right to others. In our daily life, the daytime is considered Yang; the later part of the evening is considered Yin. However, the early evening, when we are still active, is considered Yang, and later evening, when we are sleeping, is considered Yin. Your back is considered Yang and your front is considered Yin. Nevertheless, even as your back is considered Yang, it still has Yin and Yang. Your upper back is considered Yang and your lower back is considered Yin. This also helps us understand that there is good in bad, and there is bad in good.

In disease and healing, understanding the Yin-Yang theory is a large part of the practice of Traditional Chinese Medicine. A balance between the Yin organ network and the Yang organ network of the body characterizes the body in a healthy state; an unhealthy state is characterized by an imbalance between the Yin and the Yang organ networks in the body. Any excess or deficiency in the body could cause imbalance or disharmony. Sometimes both symptoms can be complicated. For instance, "hot" and "cold" can be present at the same time in different parts of the body, or at different times of the day. Chinese doctors use the Yin-Yang philosophy to diagnose and treat their patients. If an organ is weak, we use strengthening methods; if the organ is in excess, we use reduction methods. If a person has too much dampness, we use dry methods; if the person has stagnation, we use dispersion methods. If the person has too many mind activities going on, we use calming methods. If the person has too much heat, we use cooling methods, etc. If Chinese doctors work against this principle, a patient's condition would worsen.

When Yin and Yang are equal, this is the state of balanced health, or good health.

Five Elements Theory

The Five Elements theory emerged from observation of the various groups of dynamic processes, functions, and characteristics in the natural world. Everything that happens in the universe is regulated by different movements of energy. These five movements of energy form an elaborate system of mutual interaction and influence, and reference to one movement of energy is a reference to all because they are functionally interrelated and dependent on each other. The Five Elements phenomena are also seen in the human body. Energies in the universe and in our bodies are always interacting and affecting one another, simultaneously rising up, sinking down, expanding, solidifying, and connecting.

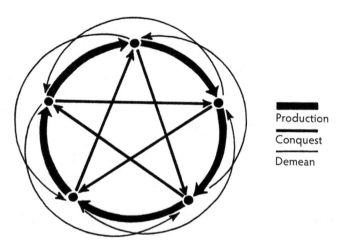

Production
Conquest
Demean

Five Elements

Each element is seen as corresponding to both the natural world and the human body. Each is linked with a season, a climate, a taste, a color, a sound, an emotion, an odor, a movement, a sense organ, a body part, Yang organs, and Yin organs. In Chinese medicine, this theory has had considerable influence in physiology, pathology, diagnosis, treatment, and pharmacology. Discussing organs such as the lungs, heart, liver, kidney, spleen, and so on is not the same as discussing the anatomical organs in our body. The words are intended to describe things from more of a general functional aspect, though it does not necessarily describe that organ's specific function, but more a set of influences.

The Five Elements are Wood, Fire, Earth, Metal and Water.

- Wood: growing, flexible, rooted, and strong.
- Fire: dry, hot, ascending, and moving.
- Earth: productive, fertile, potential for growth.
- Metal: cutting, hard, and conducting.
- Water: wet, cool, descending, flowing, and yielding.

Wood: growing, flexible, rooted, and strong. The season that corresponds with wood is spring; the color is green; the emotion is anger; and the sound is shouting. Wood energy is expansive, exhilarant, and explosive. It is associated with vigor and youth, growth and development. In TCM anatomy and physiology, wood is related to liver, (the element wood regulates the Liver and Gallbladder Meridians). The liver, which is associated with the muscles and tendons, stores the blood, maintains the free flow of Qi (energy), and controls human emotions.

Fire: dry, hot, ascending, and moving. The season that corresponds with fire is summer; the color is red; the emotions joy and happiness; and the sound is laughing. Fire energy is most energetic in the Yang phase of the cycle. It has stable heat and warmth, is upbeat, and flourishes in all activities. It is associated with love and compassion, generosity and joy, openness and abundance. In TCM anatomy and physiology, the fire is related to the heart, houses the mind, dominates the blood and vessels; the heart energy is associated with mind activity. The fire element also regulates Small Intestine, Pericardium, and Triple Warmer Meridians.

Earth: productive, fertile, potential for growth. The season that corresponds with earth is Indian summer; the color is yellow; the emotion is sympathy; and the sound is singing. Earth energy is fertile, nourishing, and vital. It provides a sense of ease, well-being, and completeness. In TCM anatomy and physiology, the earth is related to the spleen and stomach. The spleen governs transportation and transformation, which relates to digestion (absorption and metabolism). The spleen keeps blood in the vessels and prevents internal bleeding.

Metal: cutting, hard, and conducting. The season that corresponds with metal is autumn; the color is white; the emotion associated with metal is grief, and the sound is weeping. The metal energy is to condense, contract, and draw inward for accumulation and storage. In TCM anatomy and physiology, the metal energy relates to the lungs; it dominates Qi (vital energy) and controls the breath. The lungs are related to the skin, nose, and upper respiratory immune system. The metal element regulates the Lung and Large Intestine Meridians.

Water: wet, cool, descending, flowing, and yielding. The season that corresponds with water is winter; the color is blue to black; the emotion is fear; and the sound is groaning. Water energy is condensed, conserved, and stored. It contains great potential of power awaiting release. In TCM anatomy and physiology, water is related to the kidney. The kidney stores Jing (essence) and dominates human development, reproduction, sexuality, and water metabolism. It is related to bone, bone marrow, the brain, and hair. The water element regulates the Kidney and Bladder Meridians.

•••❖•••

The ancient Chinese gained the knowledge of the nature of the Five Elements through long observation of natural phenomena and ascribed certain values to them. Thus, there is an ancient saying from the early history of Traditional Chinese Medicine:

> "Wood (tree or timber) is the bending and the straightening," having the characteristics of growth, support, and effusion (upward and outward movement). The related organ energy is the liver.

"Fire is the flaming upward," having the quality of heat and upward motion. The related organ energy is the heart.

"Earth is the sowing and reaping," representing the planting and harvesting of crops and the bringing forth of phenomena. The related organ energy is the spleen.

"Metal is the working of change," having the qualities of purification, elimination, and reform. The related organ energy is the lungs.

"Water is the moistening and descending to low places," having the qualities of moistening, downward movement, and coldness. The related organ energy is the kidney.

Five Elements (or Five Phases) theory is based on an understanding of the nature of these qualities, attributed to all phenomena in the universe. The interaction of the five phases explains the nature of all phenomena. In Chinese medicine, the internal organs, body tissue, sense and other organs, emotions, and even medicinal properties are all categorized according to the phases.

It is not easy to understand the Five Elements theory completely. It requires the time necessary to study and observe nature and humans. The table below shows the relationships between humans and nature. The table should help you to understand how close humans and nature are, and give you some knowledge of disease prevention. For instance, in the spring, when liver energy is unstable, it is easy to have emotional change. In addition, a person who has a liver energy problem, the color green can be therapeutic. A person who has blocked liver energy is prone to tendonitis, so that precautions should be taken. Liver energy stagnation can make a person angry easy, and sometimes nasty.

Table Five Element Categorization of Phenomena

Item	Wood	Fire	Earth	Metal	Water
Season	Spring	Summer	Indian Summer	Autumn	Winter
Weather/ environmental factors	Wind	Heat	Dampness	Dryness	Cold
Direction	East	South	Center	West	North
Development	Birth	Growth	Maturity	Withdrawal	Dormancy
Color	Green	Red	Yellow	White	Blue/Black
Flavor	Sour	Bitter	Sweet	Acrid	Salty
Solid organ	Liver	Heart	Spleen	Lung	Kidney
Hollow organ	Gallbladder	Small Intestine	Stomach	Large Intestine	Bladder
Sense organ	Eyes	Tongue	Mouth	Nose	Ears
Tissue	Sinew, tendon	Vessels	Flesh	Hair, skin	Bone
Emotional activity	Anger	Joy and happiness	Sympathy	Sorrow/ grief	Fear
Sound	Shouting	Laughing	Singing	Weeping	Groaning
Time of day	11A.M.-3A.M.	11A.M.-3P.M.	7A.M.-11A.M.	3A.M.-7A.M.	3P.M.-7P.M.

The Five Elements are constantly interacting with, engendering, and restraining each other to achieve balance. Engendering denotes the principle whereby each phase nurtures, produces, and benefits another specific phase. Restraining refers to the principle by which each phase constrains another phase.

Arranged in cyclic form, the engendering relationships and restraining cycles are shown on the next page with their correspondences to the viscera.

The motions of engendering and restraining posit a conception of the natural world as a united whole made up of interrelated parts. *The Illustrated Supplement to the Categorized Canon (Lei Jing Tu Yi)* states:

> "The dynamic of creation cannot be without engendering or restraining;
> without engendering, there is no way by which things may arise, and with-
> out restraining, things may become unduly powerful and cause harm."

As you can see, all organs are interrelated. If any one organ has either weakness or excess, this engendering and restraining function would be lost. Therefore, the body would have various symptoms and illnesses. This is why we say that Chinese medicine is a holistic health medicine.

TCM uses a system of interrelationships between the Five Elements to understand how the various processes of the body support and control each other. Because of these interrelationships, when one of the organs and its associated element is out of balance, the other elements are eventually affected. This imbalance will manifest with many different signs and symptoms in the individual. The imbalance may show in the facial color, the sound of the voice, a rash on the skin, a change in the emotional state, a change of appetite, the sourness in certain parts of the body, as well as disharmony in the functioning of the connected organs. There are many different signs of disharmony. Some dysfunctions of the internal organs may have the same symptoms and can therefore be easily misdiagnosed. The experienced TCM doctor will use all of the information to make a clear diagnosis, determine which organ is the main cause of disharmony, and what other organ needs strengthening or unblocking.

Meridians and Energy Channels

Meridians, or channels, are energy highways that carry Qi, blood, Jing, and Jin Yie (body fluids) around the body. In ancient times, the Chinese discovery of meridians was based on how human healing related to the external injury: the injury in the external body would cause internal healing. This phenomenon was the beginning of the meridian system. Western scientists have found that meridians are difficult to identify because they do not correspond directly to nerve or blood circulation pathways. The meridian system is an energy pathway that connects all parts of the body. Some Chinese researchers believe that meridians are located throughout the body's connective tissue; others do not believe Qi exists at all, never mind the meridians. Such differences of opinion have made Chinese medicine a

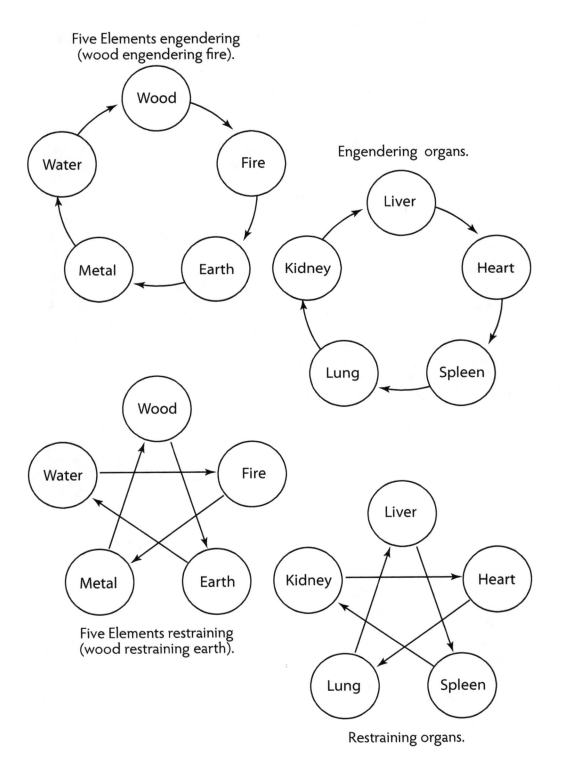

Five Elements engendering
(wood engendering fire).

Engendering organs.

Five Elements restraining
(wood restraining earth).

Restraining organs.

source of scientific controversy. Over the years, I have seen many patients feeling better and gaining great benefits after TCM care and have a high level of confidence in its healing effectiveness. A simple explanation of the existence of meridians can be had by asking the following question: Why do we feel so good after yawning when we wake up in the morning? When we yawn, we are stretching the whole body; we are actually stretching all meridians, opening the pathways, and helping energy flow better. Once energy is flowing better, our blood circulation is better, too (energy drives blood). This, in turn, allows our brains to receive more oxygen and that makes us feel alert, good, and relaxed. Our body parts receive more oxygen, so our body feels relaxed and comfortable after yawning.

There are 14 main meridians. Branching from them is a network of other smaller channels, called collaterals. Each main meridian is connected to one of the organs and travels along its own route within the body. For example, the Heart Meridian travels in a pathway from the heart itself to the armpit and down the inside of the arm to the little finger. This explains why someone with a heart problem often has a tingling feeling running down the arm to the little finger. If someone has a stomach problem, the acupuncturist will often insert needles on the points on the leg, because the Stomach Meridian goes through the leg. An understanding of how the meridian system works and where it travels can be very helpful in self-care at home. For instance, if you have a headache, just massaging the meridian and points that go through the area with pain would help you relieve the headache. A patient once told me that on one occasion when she had stomach pain; she did a five-minute self-massage on the area related to the stomach, thus relieving the pain. She did not need medication, and she was able to provide a little healing technique on herself.

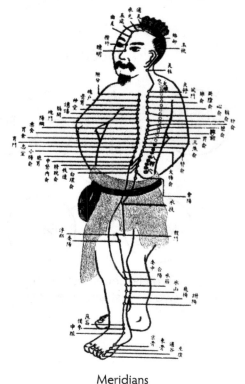

Meridians

Sometimes you may feel sore spots on your body or legs without having had any specific injury, and you might wonder why. Knowledge of TCM will help you understand that you no doubt have some blockage in your internal organs or energy circulation system. Alternatively, when you are not feeling well, you might find some sensitive spot on your body. These sensitive spots would be the "windows" that a TCM doctor would be looking for to find the signs of blockage or imbalance. These spots would also be the focus points for a practitioner to perform appropriate therapy.

Both physical and mental trauma can cause blockages in the meridian pathways; and in turn, meridian blockages can cause a physical and mental illness. The TCM practitioner always sees a person as a whole, which is an important part of the TCM practice.

The 14 major meridian and thousands of collaterals in the body traverse all parts of the body. There are six meridians in the arms (three Yin and three Yang), and six meridians in the legs (three Yin and three Yang). The meridians are the main route of energy travel, and they are deeper than collaterals. The collaterals are smaller routes for energy travel; they are shallower in the body than meridians.

Arm Meridians:
    Lung Meridian (Yin)
    Pericardium Meridian (Yin)
    Heart Meridian (Yin)
    Large Intestine Meridian (Yang)
    Triple Burner Meridian (Yang)
    Small Intestine Meridian (Yang)
Leg Meridians:
    Spleen Meridian (Yin)
    Liver Meridian (Yin)
    Kidney Meridian (Yin)
    Stomach Meridian (Yang)
    Gallbladder Meridian (Yang)
    Bladder Meridian (Yang)
Central Meridians:
    Governing Meridian (Yang)
    Conception Meridian (Yin)

Lung Meridian (Yin)

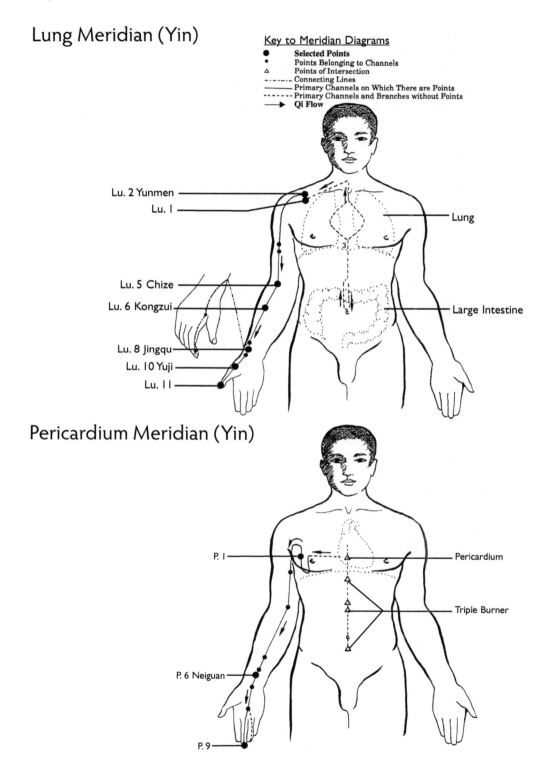

Key to Meridian Diagrams
- ● **Selected Points**
- • **Points Belonging to Channels**
- △ **Points of Intersection**
- –·–·– **Connecting Lines**
- ——— **Primary Channels on Which There are Points**
- – – – **Primary Channels and Branches without Points**
- → **Qi Flow**

Lu. 2 Yunmen
Lu. 1
Lung
Lu. 5 Chize
Lu. 6 Kongzui
Large Intestine
Lu. 8 Jingqu
Lu. 10 Yuji
Lu. 11

Pericardium Meridian (Yin)

P. 1
Pericardium
Triple Burner
P. 6 Neiguan
P. 9

Heart Meridian (Yin)

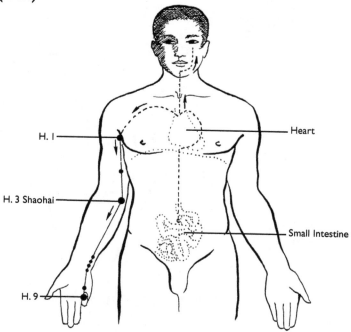

H. I

H. 3 Shaohai

H. 9

Heart

Small Intestine

Large Intestine Meridian (Yang)

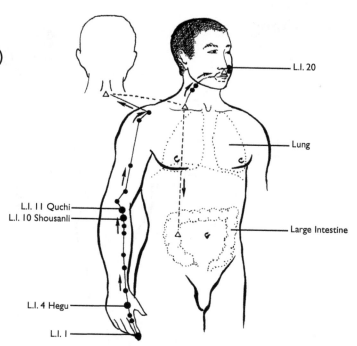

L.I. 20

Lung

L.I. 11 Quchi
L.I. 10 Shousanli

Large Intestine

L.I. 4 Hegu

L.I. I

Triple Burner
Meridian (Yang)

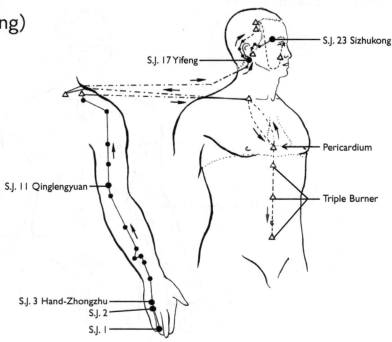

S.J. 23 Sizhukong

S.J. 17 Yifeng

Pericardium

Triple Burner

S.J. 11 Qinglengyuan

S.J. 3 Hand-Zhongzhu
S.J. 2
S.J. 1

Small Intestine
Meridian (Yang)

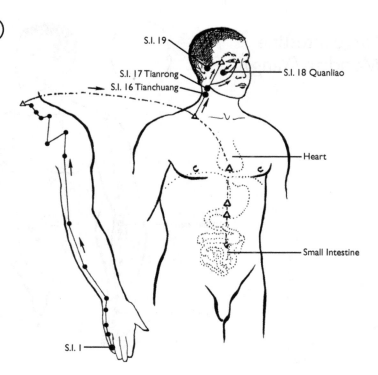

S.I. 19

S.I. 17 Tianrong

S.I. 18 Quanliao

S.I. 16 Tianchuang

Heart

Small Intestine

S.I. 1

Spleen Meridian (Yin)

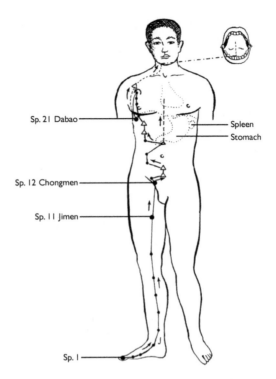

Sp. 21 Dabao

Spleen
Stomach

Sp. 12 Chongmen

Sp. 11 Jimen

Sp. 1

Liver Meridian (Yin)

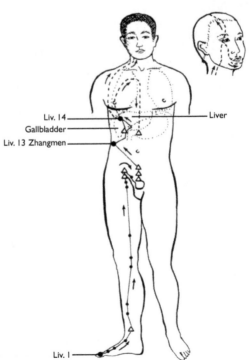

Liv. 14

Liver

Gallbladder

Liv. 13 Zhangmen

Liv. 1

Kidney Meridian (Yin)

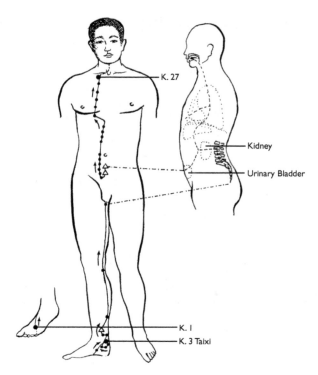

K. 27

Kidney

Urinary Bladder

K. 1

K. 3 Taixi

Stomach Meridian (Yang)

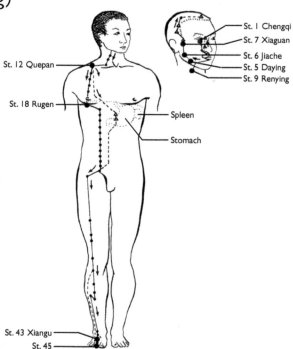

St. 1 Chengqi
St. 7 Xiaguan
St. 6 Jiache
St. 5 Daying
St. 9 Renying

St. 12 Quepan

St. 18 Rugen

Spleen

Stomach

St. 43 Xiangu
St. 45

Gallbladder Meridian (Yang)

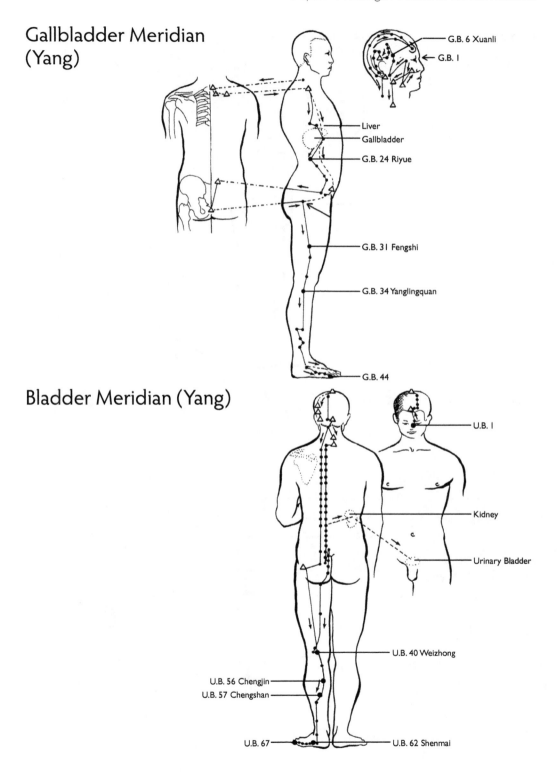

G.B. 6 Xuanli
G.B. 1
Liver
Gallbladder
G.B. 24 Riyue
G.B. 31 Fengshi
G.B. 34 Yanglingquan
G.B. 44

Bladder Meridian (Yang)

U.B. 1
Kidney
Urinary Bladder
U.B. 40 Weizhong
U.B. 56 Chengjin
U.B. 57 Chengshan
U.B. 67
U.B. 62 Shenmai

Governing
\Meridian (Yang)

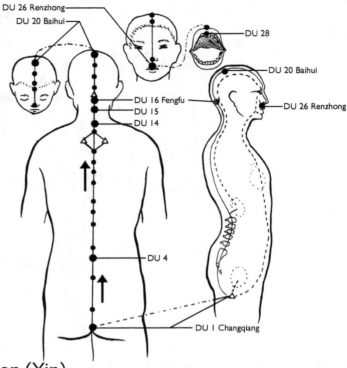

Conception Meridian (Yin)

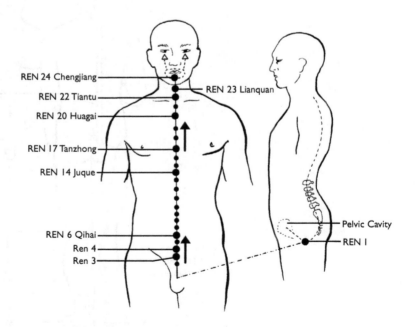

Each meridian relates to a specific organ. For example, the Lung Meridian is related to the lung; the Heart Meridian is related to the heart. However, all meridians are interrelated. One weak organ could affect other organs. If the Kidney Meridian is blocked, eventually the Lung Meridian will be affected. These meridians also have partner meridians, the solid organ (lung, heart, spleen, liver, and kidney) / hollow organ (Large Intestine, Small Intestine, Stomach, Gallbladder, and Bladder.

Lung (solid) Meridian / Large Intestine (hollow) Meridian
Pericardium (special) Meridian / Triple burner (special) Meridian
Heart (solid) Meridian / Small Intestine (hollow) Meridian
Spleen (solid) Meridian / Stomach (hollow) Meridian
Liver (solid) Meridian / Gallbladder (hollow) Meridian
Kidney (solid) Meridian / Bladder (hollow) Meridian

The function of a solid organ is to produce and store the essence; the function of a hollow organ is to decompose food and convey waste. These partner organs work closely together in maintaining normal functions of the body. If the hollow organ is weak and not corrected, in time, the partner solid organ might soon become weak as well. In addition, if the solid organ is weak and not corrected in time, the partner hollow organ might soon become weak as well.

Meridian Pathways

Even though the meridians follow a specific route in the body, they also go through the entire body, traversing through all of its parts.

- The three arm Yin meridians go from the chest to the hand, which is why we treat the hand and arm points to help relieve and heal lung disease.
- The three arm Yang meridians go from the hand to the head, which is why we treat the hand points to help to relieve headaches.
- The three leg Yin meridians go from the foot and through the leg to the chest. We use leg or foot points to treat liver or spleen problems.
- The three leg Yang meridians go from the head going through the torso and the leg to the foot, which is why we sometimes treat the leg points to help migraines.

All TCM therapists must know the meridians very well. They must also know the meridian pathways as well as their relationships with internal organs. Otherwise, the therapy would be ineffective. For instance, if you have a headache, the therapist should know which meridian blockage causes the type of headache you have. A blockage in the Stomach Meridian can cause a headache; a blockage in the Bladder Meridian can also cause a headache, as does a blockage in the Liver Meridian. If the therapist treats the wrong meridian or organ, the headache will not go away. A complete understanding of the theory of TCM makes for a better practitioner. Sometimes patients do not get results from the acupuncture treatment offered by one practitioner; this does not mean that acupuncture does not work. Rather, the patient should try a different practitioner. Patients have told me that although they had tried acupuncture elsewhere that did not work. However, they improved after treatments in our office. Other patients have told me the diagnosis by the last practitioner they had visited, but a reevaluation showed that the original diagnosis was incorrect.

TCM therapists must also know human anatomy and physiology well to help them increase their knowledge of the correct healing methods.

Characteristics of meridians:

- Connects inside/outside the body
- Connects all limbs and body
- Transports energy, essence, and blood
- Nurtures the entire body
- Defends against outside pathogens
- Protects the body from sickness

Internal Organ System of TCM (Zhang Fu)

In Chinese medicine, the term "internal organs" serves as functional terminology, a point of reference, although it is loosely based on anatomy and physiology. It does not refer exactly to the anatomical organs in the body. The term Zhang Fu is a collective name for the various Yin and Yang organs identified in TCM. It is the collection of different body functions. The Yin organ is called a Zhang organ, or solid organ, as the organ itself can be said to be solid. The Yang organ is called a Fu organ, or hollow organ as the organ itself is hollow. Each organ is considered to have its own set of functions, but these functions have a far wider scope than the purely physiological functions described in Western medicine and anatomy.

The Zhang organs consist of the five solid (Yin) organs. They are:

- Liver
- Heart
- Spleen
- Lungs
- Kidneys

In general, TCM considers the Zhang organs, which reside deeper within the body, are involved with the manufacture, storage, and regulation of the fundamental substances. For example, the heart stores and manages blood; the lung governs Qi; and the kidney stores Jing or Essence. Each Zhang organ also connects to a sensory organ, and they have an associated spiritual aspect. For example, the liver connects to the eye and is associated with mood. Zhang organs affect each other. If one organ is sick, it will eventually affect other organs. When a person is in a bad mood, he or she will feel something in the chest or stomach, which is said to feel like a lump in the body. This is called a blockage or stagnation of Qi. If this stagnation continues over the long term, his or her liver energy could become blocked. Consequently, other organs would develop problems. If this imbalance lasts too long, cancer or problems in the heart, lungs, spleen, and kidneys could develop.

The Fu organs consist of the six hollow (Yang) organs. They are:

- Gallbladder
- Small Intestine
- Stomach
- Large Intestine
- Bladder
- San Jiao or Triple Burner (there is no corresponding organ system in Western physiology or anatomy); it is a functional aspect of the body.

In general, Fu organs are closer to the surface of the body and have the functions of receiving, separating and transmitting, distributing, and excreting body substances. The Zhang organs have a close relationship to the Fu organs, so they affect each other when in disharmony. As noted before, the spleen is related to the stomach, the heart is related to the small intestine, the lung is related to the large intestine, the liver is related to the gallbladder, and the kidney is related to the bladder.

When a person has a respiratory problem, he or she most likely is low in lung energy. At the same time, he or she might experience a bowel problem, either diarrhea or constipation or other bowel symptoms. This is because the lungs and the large intestine are related as a Zhang and Fu organ pair. On the other hand, if you develop a bowel problem, eventually your lung energy will be affected. Not only do the correlated organs affect each other, but also if the disharmony lasts long term, other or all organs that have no direct relationship may also be affected. In this case, the person's illness becomes quite severe. The prognosis might be poor, and long-term treatment (even lifelong treatment) might be necessary. A patient suffering from long-term respiratory problems most likely also has weak kidney energy: Not only would he lose control of the bladder, but he would also exhibit other symptoms such as fatigue, decreased memory, body aches, and so on.

For these reasons, we should not wait too long before seeking treatment for illness, and not let the illness progress so far that other organ energies become affected. We should take care of any disharmony as soon as possible. This has always been an important principle in Chinese medicine.

The Vital Substances

TCM views the human body as an energy system in which various substances interact with each other to create the physical organism. The basic substances in the human body are Qi, blood, Jing (essence) and Jin Yie (body fluids).

Qi: Qi is translated as energy or vital energy, or life force. The word Qi has many meanings in Chinese. It is gas, air, breath, smell, weather, manner, spirit, anger, be bullied, and vital energy. As you can see, none of the above is visible, but all are related to the air or oxygen, and mental activity. In this book, Qi refers to vital energy as related to human health and vitality.

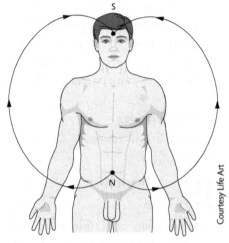

Human energy field.

Qi is the energy that underlies everything in the universe. In the Chinese character for Qi, 氣 we can see the rice 米 is under the air 气. When it comes to human energy, there would be no Qi without either rice (or food) and air.

Qi refers to the various types of bioenergy associated with human health and vitality. Qi is associated with the lung through breathing. Breathing extracts external energy from air and blends it in the bloodstream with the internal energy extracted by digestion from food and water. The resulting blend is the basis for human energy, metabolism, and immune function. Qi is present internally and externally and controls the function of all parts of the body.

There are many different kinds of energy in the universe, electricity, solar energy, nuclear energy, hydroelectric energy, magnetic energy. Modern life is based on energy. Without this energy, we would still be living a primitive life. Energy in the air helps plants and animal grow better and remain healthy; energy surrounds buildings and brings good luck and healthy living; energy in food supplies nutrition to the body, and energy in our brain creates a fresh outlook.

Qi keeps us moving and functioning, keeps us warm, and protects us against sickness. Everything we do involves Qi. Walking, eating, laughing, crying, playing sports, working, hiking, and writing are all related to Qi. With good Qi, you will be healthy and happy, work more efficiently, and be more creative. If you have bad or poor Qi, you will be unhappy and unhealthy, your life will tend to be more difficult, your work will tend to be hard, and you may have more complaints that are physical. Qi affects our life everyday. We cannot see the Qi in the body, but we can feel it. Just as we cannot see electricity in the wire, we sure feel it if we touch a hot wire. Qi is very important in the body and in life, but how many people really pay attention to Qi? How many doctors are really examining the quality of their patients' Qi?

Blood: In TCM, the term blood does not describe exactly the same substance as its counterpart in Western medicine. In TCM, not only does blood include the Western concept of blood that carries oxygen and nutrients, but it also means the fluid that nourishes and moisturizes the body and assists in the flow of Qi. Additionally, blood aids in the development of clear and stable thought processes. Disharmonies of the blood include deficient blood, which typically leads to a pale complexion, dry skin, and dizziness. Stagnant blood can cause sharp and intense pain, or even the development of tumors. "Heat in the blood" is a condition that causes bleeding symptoms such as uterine hemorrhage or nosebleeds. Other conditions, such as chronic pain, arthritis, fibromyalgia, and other disorders, develop when both the Qi and blood are stagnant. Qi and blood have a very close relationship. If there is problem in Qi circulation, blood circulation and vise versa are soon affected.

Jing (Essence): It is crucial to the development of the individual throughout life. It is inherited at birth, is stored in the kidneys, and allows us to develop from childhood to adulthood, and then into old age. It governs growth, reproduction, and development, promotes kidney Qi, and works with Qi to help protect the body from external pathogens. Any developmental disorder, such as learning difficulties and physical abilities in children, may be due to a deficiency of Jing from birth. Other disorders such as infertility, poor memory, a tendency to get sick or catch colds, and allergies may also be due to a Jing deficiency. Jing has a very close relationship to the Western term "gene," a genetic material.

Jin Yie (Body fluids): In addition to blood, they are considered the organic liquids that moisten and lubricate the body. They are similar to what Western physiology calls body fluids. These fluids moisten and nourish the skin, muscles, hair, joints, brain, spine, and bone marrow. Deficiency in body fluids can lead to various forms of dehydration such as dry skin and constipation. If fluids accumulate and become stuck (in Western terminology, this is described as water retention), this situation can lead to problems of dampness and build-up of phlegm. The condition may manifest such symptoms as lethargy and a feeling of heaviness and bloat in the body. Women often experience these symptoms during the days leading up to their menstrual periods.

Disharmony or Imbalance

My patients often ask me questions like, "Why do I have this disease? What was the cause?" "Why do I have it now as I never had it before?" Understanding the cause of illness is the first step in preventing illness. Diseases often spring from multiple sources that affect our energy and immune system. TCM divides the causes of disharmony into three main areas: Internal Causes, External Causes, and Miscellaneous Causes.

Internal Causes: Internal causes are illnesses caused by emotional change, principally stress. We live in a stressful society and have stressful lifestyles; we often forget how to relax. We feel we have to be busy all the time. Our children are very busy, and they have a lot of stress, too. Many of them also have emotional problems. When the mind is overly stimulated, and the body is overused, it affects our nervous and hormone systems, leading to emotional imbalance. There is good stress (positive) and bad stress (negative) that affects us every day. We understand that the bad stress can cause many problems, but we do not realize that good stress causes problems, too. We assume good stress should be healthy, but this is not always true. Good stress is only considered healthy if it does not cause emotional problems or emotionally extreme behavior. Good stress that leads to emotional extremes may also lead to illness, which is not good at all!

The emotions that are related to disease due to internal causes include anger, sadness, worry, fear, joy, pensiveness, and shock, which are usually referred to as the Seven Emotions. From the Western viewpoint, we could say these are emotional changes

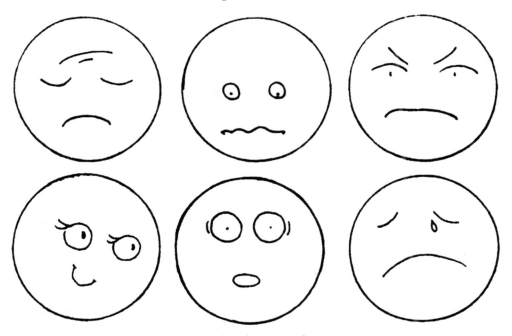

Emotions related to internal causes.

caused by stress. While these emotions are normal and healthy responses to the many situations we encounter in daily life, they can cause disease when they are intense or prolonged, or if they are not expressed or acknowledged over long periods of time. In other words, if these emotions are too extreme or last too long, they can cause problems.

One of my patients told me several years ago that her neighbor's husband died at his 50th birthday party. Nobody could believe that experiencing so much joy could be a problem. Anything extreme or excessive can cause problems. Consider how you would feel if you lost a job you needed for supporting your family. Would you be able to sleep at night? Would you have enough energy in the morning? Imagine if your boss accused you of something in which you were not involved; how would you feel? Would you sleep soundly that night? Would you be happy at work? What would happen to your health as a result? This is why we say high stress can cause extreme emotional changes, consequently causing physical problems. Understanding Chinese medicine and the Daoist philosophy can help you improve personal stress management, and you will become more emotionally stable. You would become more likely to remain balanced no matter what unexpected events may happen to you, which in turn helps prevent health problems.

> I had three people tell me about deaths that occurred in a positive atmosphere: a man died at his 50th birthday surprise party; an elderly woman died at her 80th birthday party; a singer died on stage while he was performing. On the other hand, we know from our own experience how tired we are after we host a big party. We had a good time, but we felt very tired afterward, due to the enormous work; we needed several days to recuperate.

From the perspective of the theory of Five Elements, the first complete book in Chinese medicine *Huang Di Nei Jing*, known in English as *The Yellow Emperor's Classic of Internal Medicine* written over 2,000 years ago, describes the way that the five emotions affect specific organs:

Anger affects the liver
Overjoy affects the heart
Worry affects the lungs
Pensiveness affects the spleen
Fear or fright affects the kidneys

Over time, other Chinese doctors discovered more relationships between emotions and the organs:

Anger affects the liver
Overjoy affects the heart
Worry affects the lungs and spleen
Pensiveness affects the spleen
Sadness affects the lungs and heart

Fear or fright affects the kidneys
Shock affects the kidneys and heart

According to the classic study of Chinese medicine, these are called the Seven Emotions and are considered harmful to the human body and mind.

In modern society, with its fast-paced lifestyle, there are more emotions involved in our life that can cause an imbalance of human energy. Thus, the list of emotions could be expanded as follows:

Anger (and frustration and resentment) affects the liver
Overjoy affects the heart
Worry affects the lungs and spleen
Pensiveness affects the spleen
Sadness (and grief) affects the lungs and heart
Fear or fright affects the kidneys
Shock affects the kidneys and heart
Love affects the heart
Hatred affects the heart and liver
Craving affects the heart
Guilt affects kidneys and heart

The "simple question" (from over 2000 years ago) in Chapter 23 of *The Yellow Emperor's Classic of Internal Medicine* mentions:

"The Heart houses the Mind,
the Lungs houses the Corporeal Soul,
the Liver houses the Ethereal Soul,
the Spleen houses the Intellect and
the Kidneys house the Will-Power."

Chapter 9 reveals that:

"The Heart is the root of life and the origin of the Mind... the Lungs are the root of Qi and the dwelling place of the Corporeal Soul... the Kidneys are the root of sealed storage (essence) and the dwelling of Will-Power... the Liver is the root of harmonization and the residence of the Ethereal Soul..."

All of the organs are related to the functions of the human mind and emotion. The organs that are related to depression are the heart and liver. The heart relates to your mind, and the liver relates to your emotions. Other organs can affect the heart and liver. In Chinese medicine, the organs connect in a network in which the organs support each other. It is important to correct each organ's imbalance to prevent future problems in other organs.

External Causes: External causes that create disharmony are mostly related to climatic conditions. There are six of these conditions, usually known as the six pathogenic factors or the Six Outside Evils. They are wind, cold, damp, fire/heat, dryness, and summer heat. Different climate conditions occur during each season and we usually adapt to them as they come and go. However, extremes of weather, such as a very cold winter or an unseasonably warm spell in winter, make us more vulnerable to the effects of that climatic condition and consequently more vulnerable to becoming ill. In addition, people whose underlying or reserve energy is weak are more vulnerable to the effects of climatic conditions than those who have a strong constitution. Many years ago, a patient insisted that catching cold is due to a viral infection, not due to the weather change. I know his statement is based on knowledge that he gained from his doctor, but he did not understand that the interior landscape of the body is the key in human health. The balanced or harmonized body would have a good immune function, would be able to fight against any microorganism, and able to adapt any climatic change. When the weather changes in the extreme and you are not dressed properly, this would change your interior landscape, thus affecting the Yin-Yang balance in the body. The changes cause an imbalance in the energy system, so your immune function becomes weak. Therefore, you are prone to infection from a virus or bacteria, and you could become sick easily. That is why the Chinese say catch a cold, not a virus.

Other external causes are environmental factors, such as exposure to chemicals, bacteria, radiation, pollutants, and microorganisms. These factors can cause imbalances in the body energy that lead to illness.

Miscellaneous Causes: Miscellaneous causes include overwork, inappropriate exercise, poor or wrong diet, abnormal sexual activity, and physical trauma. TCM teaches that these factors can have a profound influence on our bodies. For example, too much physical work can impair Qi; mental activity can damage the spleen; too much anger will impair the liver; and someone who works outdoors is more liable to be at risk from microorganisms including bacteria, viruses, parasites, etc. Outdoor workers are also easily affected by climate changes. Various injuries not corrected in time will make the body more vulnerable to the outside pathogens. Excessive sexual activity is thought to impair kidney energy, especially kidney Jing (essence). Mental attitude can also be a factor in energy imbalance. A strongly negative attitude can cause many problems and blockages in the organ system, especially affecting the liver and heart (remember, the TCM concept of liver or heart is not the same as the anatomical organs known as the liver and heart). In many cases, disease is caused from multiple factors.

The important lesson of Chinese healing is to do things in moderation, neither too much nor too little. Chinese natural healing is about the balance of Yin and Yang. If your body is balanced, you will not only be healthy, but also happy. This is the secret of health and longevity, which the Chinese have known for centuries.

TCM Diagnostic Methods

Chinese diagnoses are not made easily, and it takes a long time for TCM practitioners to learn how to make correct diagnoses. Only an experienced and dedicated practitioner can make correct diagnoses. If the diagnosis is incorrect, treatment will not be as effective, or sometimes may even make the condition worse. Some patients read a TCM book and feel they can make a diagnosis themselves, and then go to a store to buy some herbs. Self-help should be encouraged, but is not recommended if you have a serious medical issue. As a layperson, you should not tell the TCM practitioner how to do their job. Your training is far less than the doctor-practitioner's training.

A patient suffering from a major back problem came to see me; he told me that his Spleen Meridian was blocked. After I examined him, I found that his diagnosis was wrong. His main problems were in the liver and kidneys, as well as blockages in the Bladder Meridian. He might have read some books, or gone to other therapists who were not fully trained in TCM. The patient did not understand TCM thoroughly, which was why his condition was not improving.

TCM is quite a complicated science because many overlapping symptoms can cause confusion in diagnoses, even to practitioners. When patients do not find relief from TCM care, it might be because the wrong diagnosis led to ineffective treatment. Oftentimes thorough knowledge of TCM is not enough; you need to know about human anatomy, physiology, biochemistry, characteristics of illness, and clinical study. In China, we do not have acupuncturists; we have acupuncture doctors, most of who work in hospitals and clinics, with fewer in private practice. Very often, the doctors who practice Western medicine refer patients to TCM doctors to relieve symptoms and speed the healing process. While working in a Chinese hospital as an obstetrician/gynecologist, I was treating cancer patients with chemotherapy; however, I sometimes used acupuncture to treat the nausea caused by chemotherapy as well as Chinese herbal medicine to balance the energy and promote digestion. For anemic patients, I included Chinese herbs in their treatment that helped the body produce blood cells. In Western medicine, a doctor might often give iron for anemia. TCM doctors normally do not give iron unless we know the anemia is caused from iron deficiency. Using Chinese herbs to treat anemia has been effective for many centuries.

TCM diagnoses are very different from Western diagnoses. TCM does not use expensive equipment; instead, it relies completely on the TCM practitioner's training, experience, and knowledge. The cost of TCM health care is much less than the cost of conventional health care. Because expensive equipment is not used, TCM is also much less invasive. The effectiveness of any treatment is largely based on the accuracy of the diagnosis. The accuracy of most TCM diagnoses is between 80 and 90 percent, but there are many factors that can affect the treatment. Just as in Western medicine, TCM diagnoses can be either single or multiple. A person can have weak lungs as well as a weak stomach. We have previously mentioned that the internal organs are related to each other. In a Western diagnosis, a person can have hypertension and arthritis. The TCM practitioner should not ignore the Western diagnosis; it will often help in the overall treatment. For instance, to treat a person with anemia, the TCM practitioner can prescribe a blood tonic herb to help strengthen the blood, as well as treatment to stimulate the organ to produce more blood cells. If the patient just takes an iron pill, it might disturb other minerals used for metabolism in the body and cause other problems. Moreover, the anemia can have other causes besides a lack of iron. When doctors cannot find any problem with the patient, they should refer him or her to a TCM doctor or acupuncturist. The TCM doctor will look for a blockage on the meridian and organ system (energy system) that may not necessarily be visible in the test results. The practitioner needs to know the patient's lifestyle, diet, and working situation, which all help make the diagnosis. For instance, a diet heavy in cheese or sugar tends to cause blockages in the spleen. Cheese can cause dampness in the body; in terms of a Western medical explanation, too much cheese can cause water retention and even a weight problem.

In TCM, the diagnostic process considers four perspectives — known as the Four Examinations. These are looking, hearing and smelling, questioning, and touching.

Looking

The TCM doctor examines the patient's complexion, eyes, tongue, nails, hair, gait, stature, and affect. The Chinese doctor will also look at the patient's Shen (spirit) and Qi (energy). An experienced TCM doctor can tell right away whether your energy is weak or strong. Ten years ago, at a professional conference, I told a woman that her kidney energy was weak; she was insulted and even became angry with me. I thought I had done her a favor by giving her a free diagnosis, but I forgot about the cultural differences between people in China and those in the United States. I learned my lesson and do not diagnose people unless they have an appointment with me.

Hearing and Smelling

This involves listening to the sound of a patient's voice and breathing, and noticing the smell of the breath and skin.

In Western medicine, certain smells can be signs of illness. The severe diabetic who develops ketone acidosis has a strong smell that a doctor can recognize. Certain liver diseases can also have certain smells that help the Western doctor make the right diagnosis.

Questioning

Just as it is important in Western medicine, in TCM, listening to the patient's complaints is very important. Patients can give you valuable information, thus helping you make the right diagnosis and treatment plan. The patient's current complaints, health history, family health history, patterns of sleep, dietary habits, bowel movements, urination, sweat, physical pain, emotional status, previous surgeries or illnesses, lifestyle, exercise patterns, working conditions, and gynecological history are all necessary to collect and keep in the patient's file. This information helps the TCM practitioner figure out why the patient might have a particular illness and give proper guidance to the patient for his or her own self-care.

One time I told a student that he had a stomach problem. He was astonished and asked me how I knew. I could not tell him that it was because I smelled the certain odor that indicated a weak stomach, because in American culture, people do not like to hear someone telling them that they smell; but in China, people do not mind hearing this information. Usually, an experienced TCM practitioner can tell that the person has a weak organ from hearing or smelling. My patients often joke with me, saying, "Dr. Kuhn, you are scary, you know everything," but it is just my experience with medicine and healing.

Touching

Touching in Chinese medicine practice is very important for a correct diagnosis. Without touching, one cannot find the truth about what is causing the ailment. Similar to the way a Western doctor relies on different tests to find out what is going on in the body, the Chinese doctor relies on their hands to find out what is going on and why this person has the symptoms. Touching involves feeling the body parts to discover body temperature, body moisture, and the nature and location of the pain. Touching also involves checking the energy pathways to see if there are any blockages in the energy path. If the doctor does not know how to find these blockages, treatment will not be effective.

There is another important touching technique, called pulse diagnosis or taking the pulse. The pulse diagnosis is a rather complicated process that requires years of experience to perfect. In Western medical practice, the pulse is checked to determine its speed and rhythm, or to see if there is any pulse. In Chinese medicine, besides checking the rhythm of the pulse, the practitioner checks to determine its size, its depth, shape, and its speed as well as its organ status.

Another important touching technique is ear diagnosis. Not all Chinese doctors or acupuncturists are able to do ear diagnosis because special training is required. Similar to reflexology, this technique maps points on the body to points on the ear. Your ear has a shape similar to that of an upside-down fetus, in that the parts of the fetus' shape correlate to specific points on the ear; hence, to the patient's body. The practitioner will use a small instrument to find the points on the ear that are related to the body parts having a blockage or other problem.

The practitioners will combine other diagnostic methods to make a more accurate diagnosis. Some practitioners can perform ear therapy, called auricular acupressure, which is based on ear acupuncture. Now, the practitioners use herbs instead of needles. They put herb seeds on the ear points that related to the problems.

Touching is very important in diagnosis and making the right plan for healing. One of my patients told me a story about going to the doctor for back pain. Her doctor did not even touch her, but merely gave her pain medication. Back pain has many causes: muscle, bone, tendon, nerve, or joints. Furthermore, back pain can occur in different locations: upper back, lower back, middle back, etc. Each different cause of the pain needs the appropriate treatment. If you do not touch the patient, how can you know if the real problem is the muscle, bone, disk, or nerve? If the problem can be found by touching, the doctor or practitioner will be better able to offer the right therapy. To be a good doctor, touching with professional skill is essential.

Diagnosing a patient's condition using Traditional Chinese Medicine is not at all easy. Only experienced Chinese doctors will be able to make a clear diagnosis. Making the right diagnosis will help the practitioner to determine the appropriate treatment plan and achieve good results.

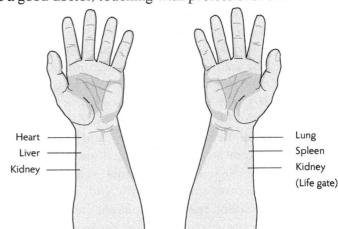

Heart
Liver
Kidney

Lung
Spleen
Kidney
(Life gate)

Palms of hands (courtesy of LifeArt)

TCM Treatments

As previously discussed, a myriad of pathogens and factors can cause illness, which cause imbalance in the body energy and immune system that makes us feel depressed and sick. In most cases, our body's healing ability can gradually help us to fight off illness. If the body becomes overpowered by sickness or it is beyond your body's ability to fight it off, the body will become weak, and energy and blood circulation will become weak and inefficient. You will experience many different symptoms to which your doctor will give a collective name, like Chronic Fatigue Syndrome or fibromyalgia, for which the doctor will prescribe medication to relieve the symptoms. Alternatively, you might experience long-term discomfort and unhappiness if the symptoms are left untreated. This is the time when you need TCM care.

TCM treatment uses various therapeutic methods to restore balance, promote energy/blood circulation, strengthen the immune system, and enhance the body's healing ability. Once your body is balanced and your immune system is intact, your organ function will stay normal, your mental status will stay clear, your emotions will stay even and relaxed. You will have less sickness, less stress, and more energy. You will also be more productive and have a better life. Your body will change physically, spiritually, and psychologically.

Disease in Western medicine is described by a specific name. If the doctor gives the condition the wrong name or misdiagnoses the disease, it will affect the healing process. In Chinese medicine, there is no individual name for a disease; rather, the status or nature of each patient's condition is described by the practitioner. Any kind of illness in Chinese medicine can be described by the categories: vacuity, excess, stagnation, imbalance, and so on. The treatment of Chinese medicine will balance these conditions in order to hasten the healing process.

Do you go to the mechanic to have your car serviced regularly (e.g., tune-ups, oil changes, alignment, and so on)? Why do you maintain your car? Of course, the answer is to have it last longer, run more smoothly, and reduce the risk of the car breaking down. What about regular service that can make your life longer, healthier, or happier? Many people pay a lot of money to fix or maintain their car, but they are not willing to spend money on the maintenance of their health. I have always believed that it is more important to maintain good health than to maintain a car.

If given by an experienced practitioner, all TCM treatments are completely natural with no side effects. TCM treatments work on the body's energy system, bringing the body to harmony and balance. Most treatments are effective, but if the TCM treatment does not work on the specific ailment, it will surely benefit other parts of the body. We call this "side benefits." Patients often come to get treatment for one problem, but, in the end, their other problems improve due to these side benefits. For example, a patient came to my office for treatment for her back pain. After getting treatments for her pain, not only was her back pain gone, but also her energy and emotional state improved as had her digestive problems. Other patients come to the office for treatment for their blood pressure problems. After their treatments their cholesterol level drops and their blood sugar becomes normal, along with improved blood pressure.

TCM treatment is considered TCM therapy. Compared with physical therapy, TCM therapy is more effective and powerful due to its unique healing system. Physical therapy and TCM used in conjunction with each other can achieve excellent healing results. More and more physical therapists refer patients to acupuncturists, Chinese doctors, or Chinese massage doctors. TCM practitioners also refer patients for physical therapy. This cooperation has proven that Western and Eastern healing work very well together. TCM helps patients recover much more quickly from various surgeries. I often see surgical patients in my office and have found that they recover much sooner than do patients without TCM care.

TCM treatments may vary depending on the nature of the ailment. How long the ailment has existed and the location of the ailment are always concerns. TCM has no side effects, but if a person has an allergy problem, he or she might have a reaction to herbs. Similarly, a nervous individual might feel worse after acupuncture treatment, which is why a nervous person should start with Chinese massage before acupuncture; or the acupuncturist should treat this person with a very gentle technique, and use fewer needles. Some people have a fear of needles, but TCM is not just about needles and acupuncture. Treatments using acupressure can do a wonderful job for those who are afraid of needles. I have had small children brought to me by their parents. The babies felt better with acupressure and Qigong healing methods, which understandably made the parent feel better. Besides acupuncture, there are many different TCM methods of treatment available. Some ailments can be helped with Chinese herbal medicine, others may have better results with acupuncture treatments, while still others get more benefits from Chinese massage therapy. Individuals may need only auricular acupressure therapy. Even practicing Chinese exercises has helped many people. A healthy diet is also a very important tool in both healing and disease prevention. Other methods of self-healing, presented later in this book, are important as well.

We should be aware that many people who come to a TCM clinic have chronic conditions that require long-term treatment. Just one or two treatments will not get rid of a problem that has persisted for many years. Many people are looking for a quick fix, but good health takes time to maintain, and a wound takes time to heal. Some people may require a lifetime of health maintenance care. People who want a quick fix tend to take medications, but if one has low tolerance to the side effects of the medication, they may develop other health problems. They then need other medication to treat the side effects. The more medication they take, the more problems they have. This does not mean we do not need medication; it means we need to use it wisely without harming our body. TCM treatments may give you quick results for some conditions, but other conditions may take treatments over a long time to produce long-lasting results. The effectiveness of the treatment is related to your lifestyle, diet, exercise, mental clarity, situations at work and at home, self discipline skills in stress management, and the features of your illness.

The longer you have had discomfort, the longer the treatment you will need; furthermore, the more skeptical you are, the less you will experience beneficial effects because you are less likely to follow the instructions for treatment at home. The less discipline you have, the less benefit you will get; and the more medication you take, the less healthy you will be. The patient's cooperation with the doctor is also an important part of the healing process.

If your energy is blocked or weak, the nutrients you take are not used or metabolized well by the body. For instance, if you have weak spleen and stomach energy, no matter how well you eat, you will still be tired and bloated because your food will not be metabolized well. If you have weak kidney energy, no matter how much calcium you take, you will still have osteoporosis because the calcium would not be deposited in the bone, so the bone will still be lacking calcium. If your energy is flowing well, you do not need to take much medicines and supplements. Your normal daily food and drink are enough to support your body's functions and metabolism. If you use medications wisely, that is, when you really need to, they work very well. Long-term use of medications not only causes side effects, but also causes other problems to the body in the future. Most medication is metabolized by the liver and eliminated through the kidney and is, therefore, toxic to the liver and kidney. In Chinese medicine, these two organs are very important in maintaining human health and longevity. In depressed patients, the liver energy is already stagnated, and their medication could only make the liver more vulnerable or weak.

> A 38-year-old patient came to me with 20 different medications and supplements he had been taking, and he told me that he was still felling terrible: low energy, stomach problems, and upper respiratory and sinus infections. I examined him with TCM methods and found that his kidney, stomach, and spleen energies were not balanced. I told him that he would not do well if he continued taking all of his medicines and supplements. After he discontinued most of them, as well as having TCM treatment for a while, he felt much better. Within three months, he became completely normal and healthy.

Acupuncture

Acupuncture is one of the oldest, most commonly used medical procedures in the world. It has become the biggest part of TCM treatment in the United States in the years since 1972 when President Nixon visited China, at which time he saw amazing results for patients during his visits to hospitals. In 1993, the U.S. Food and Drug Administration (FDA) estimated that Americans made 9 to 12 million visits per year to acupuncture practitioners and spent as much as $500 million on acupuncture treatments. Now we are seeing pain clinics, primary care doctors, orthopedic surgeons, and rheumatologists making more referrals for acupuncture treatment.

Acupuncture treatment stimulates the body's energy points to balance biochemicals such as increasing endorphins in the brain, which plays an important role in reducing pain, increasing the serotonin level that is often deficient in people who have depression and lowering the level of norepinephrine and dopamine that helps to relieve anxiety and manic conditions. Acupuncture also works on the autonomic nervous system, which influences the body's self-regulating mechanisms, thus enhancing our self-healing abilities and promoting physical and emotional well-being. It also stimulates the immune system, making immune cells more active in the body. Studies in China have shown that acupuncture treatment may alter brain chemistry by affecting the release of neurotransmitters and neurohormones in a beneficial way. Acupuncture affects the central nervous system as it is related to sensation and involuntary body functions, such as immune reactions and processes whereby a person's blood pressure, blood flow, and body temperature are

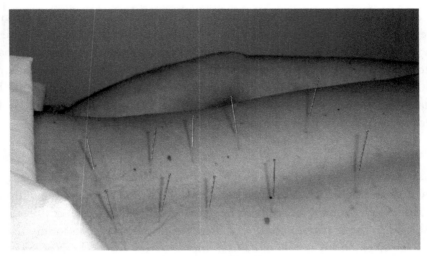

Acupuncture Needles

regulated. In China, acupuncture is used to treat cancer and reduce the side effects of chemotherapy and radiation therapy. The benefits from acupuncture for treating cancer come from an enhanced immune function, which promotes healing and helps the body to fight the cancer.

In China, many people use herbal medicine to treat their problems. Acupuncture is used for pain reduction. In the United States, acupuncture is used for an assortment of problems, including digestion, addiction, circulation, immune system weaknesses, hypertension and heart disease, chronic fatigue, emotional problems, insomnia, headache and muscle aches, arthritis, sciatica, poor vision, stroke, infertility, PMS, fibroids, asthma, back pain, and sinus and neck problems. Because many Chinese can take herbal preparations made up of leaves, minerals, seeds, roots, and all other plant parts, those who have these kinds of problems use herbal medicine more often than acupuncture, even though the herbs require cooking and do not taste good. In recent years, it seems an increased number of people in China go to acupuncture treatment and massage therapy.

Acupuncture is called needle treatment or needle therapy. The acupuncturist inserts needles of various lengths into different body points on the meridian pathway. These points are located on or join in channels or meridians; it is along these meridians that the Qi (energy) flows. You might think of Qi as a train traveling along on railroad tracks, which are the meridians, and the acupuncture points are the train stations, or the energy stations. The treatment is like opening the tracks to let the train go through.

The points are used in treatment, and are carefully chosen by the TCM practitioner to disperse any blockages or stagnations, and bring the patient's Qi and blood into balance. The stimulation from acupuncture not only activates the energy system, but also changes body chemicals and neural transmitters in the blood system and between the cells in the body. This kind of natural stimulation is safe and effective for many conditions. Patients feel sensations that have been described as heavy, tight, strong, deep ache, dull ache. If the patient feels a sharp pain, the practitioner should reinsert the needle, because the needle hit a nerve ending or a small blood vessel. Conversely, if there is no sensation at all, the needle has not been placed at the acupuncture point, making the treatment less effective. Only if the needle is inserted at the right place, will the treatment work.

Moxibustion

Moxibustion is the process whereby a dried herb is burned indirectly above the skin, above specific acupuncture points, or the herb is attached to acupuncture needles, and then burned in order to heat the needles. This procedure warms the Qi and blood in the meridian channels. Moxibustion is most commonly used when there is a requirement to expel cold and dampness from the body. Not every patient requires moxibustion. If the practitioner uses moxibustion on a patient with a heat-type physical constitution and symptoms, the problem can become worse. Moxibustion is often used with acupuncture. Moxibustion can also be used in self-care. You can ignite the Moxi-roll which is made from an herb called Ai Yie (*Artemisia argyi*), and then hold it above your skin near the problem or acupoint that relates to the problem. This self-healing method helps relieve pain and promotes circulation that helps heal the affected tissue. The patient should have some knowledge of the body's meridian system and acupuncture points, so that he or she can be instructed by the acupuncturist on how to perform the treatment.

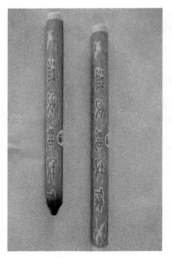
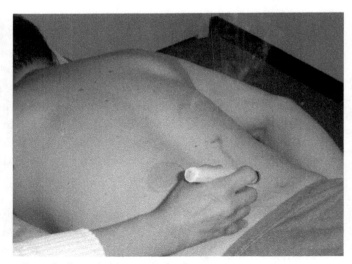

Mox-Roll, made from the Artemisia herb.

Cupping

Some Chinese practitioners like to use the cupping technique, which requires special training. Like moxibustion, the cupping technique is effective for many ailments, especially for reducing pain caused by the stagnation of Qi and blood. I have had many people come to me for treatment for back pain. Some of them were treated with the cupping technique. The cupping technique involves creating a vacuum in a cup, which is placed on the body. The airless cup is put on the skin above the area that has the stagnation and left there for about four minutes (the amount of time will vary for different patients). The technique unblocks the stagnation of Qi and blood, and patients feel better immediately. If the cupping is not tight enough, the procedure will fail. If the cupping is left on the patient's body too long, more stagnation occurs, which affirms that the TCM practitioner needs to be well trained.

In early years, practitioners used bamboo cups for treatment. Now, however, they primarily use special glass jars. The cupping treatment might leave a purple mark on the body. During the summer time, especially when you plan to go to beach, you might want to avoid the treatment altogether!

Tui Na (Chinese Massage)

This experience is my favorite, and every year that I go to China, I always make sure to have my Chinese massage.

Chinese massage, called Tui Na or An Mo, is the oldest manual, natural healing method. It was developed earlier than herbs and acupuncture. At first, humans fought against disease by using their own hands and body parts. Later they developed other natural methods for healing and disease prevention.

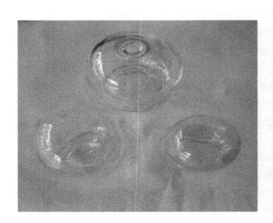
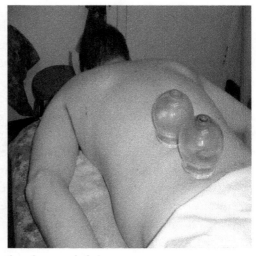

Cupping jar made from bamboo and glass.

Chinese massage is good for health maintenance as well as healing. The method was fostered by Chinese doctors in their long struggle against disease. It is based on traditional TCM theories of Qi, Blood, visceral organs, meridians, and collaterals, and is characterized by more than 20 commonly used manipulations and techniques. It includes pressing, rolling, pushing, grasping, kneading, vibrating, chopping, pinching, pulling, rubbing, and to name but a few. These techniques can be used individually or combined together. They are applied on specific acupuncture points, meridians, muscles, and skin areas with different parts of the palms and fingers and varying degrees of force. Chinese massage technique is intended to focus on the Qi rather than just using brutal force. By learning how to use the Qi, the practitioner can make the force more penetrating and activating. Patients experience good pain or enjoyable pain. The patient immediately feels looser in the muscles and joints, and more relaxed. Many people use Chinese massage as a substitute for medication and acupuncture. Chinese massage has four different massage categories: therapeutic, health maintenance, range of motion, and self-healing. At present, two more massage categories have been developed: beauty and occupational (athletic therapeutic). Sometimes herbal liquids and extracts may be required to achieve extra healing benefits.

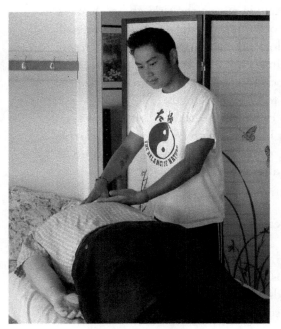

Tui Na massage.

Chinese massage is recognized as the ancestor of massage and has provided us with many benefits throughout the centuries. Europeans, Japanese, and other Asian people learned it more than a thousand years ago. Using Chinese massage as a foundation, they then developed their own specialized massage styles with their own unique character. We know them today as Swedish massage, shiatzu, and Thai massage. These massage types focused on health maintenance, whereas Chinese massage focuses on healing and improving health. Today, people from all over the world come to China to learn this unique, natural healing method. As a result, new populations become involved with this ancient art of healing.

Chinese massage is very different from Western massage. It is much more strenuous and powerful. It is deeply penetrating and goes into the acupuncture points and meridians, activating the Qi and Blood, and promoting circulation to speed the healing process.

Besides helping with many kinds of ailments, TCM massage is well known for helping with joint and muscle problems. TCM massage is used to assist internal healing, too (due to its effect on the energy channels). Chinese massage is so-called because the massage is applied chiefly to acupuncture points and meridians, which are all based on TCM theory.

In China years ago, massage therapy was usually performed by doctors in a hospital. In China now, due to increased demand, there are many training centers for massage therapists; but a massage therapist is not the same as a massage doctor who works in a hospital treating illness.

In China, most trained massage therapists perform Chinese massage more for health maintenance and focus less on treating illness, whereas the massage doctors in China work on patients primarily to relieve their ailments. To be able to treat illness, the massage therapists need to have a vast knowledge of physiology, anatomy, TCM theory, and clinical experience, including biochemistry.

Sometimes chiropractor's manipulations are also applied by Chinese massage doctors. These manipulations are clearly described in numerous Chinese massage books. Chinese massage can help heal ailments, both internal and external, and it is a good therapy for health maintenance. Chinese massage is safe and enjoyable, and Chinese patients can tolerate the manipulation. Patients may feel pain when their problems are severe; but after being treated regularly, they feel much better. Practitioners oftentimes perform various techniques, including joint movement and range of motion. Chinese massage can be applied to patients of any age including seniors and pregnant women. For children, Chinese massage can be a substitute for acupuncture. I have been using Chinese massage for pediatric care for quite a while and observed the fact that kids respond very well. Ailments that can be relieved by Chinese massage include headache, insomnia, asthma, indigestion, injury, bowel, back, and neck problems, stiffness, fibromyalgia, mild or moderate hypertension, diabetes, etc. Best of all is the good feeling that comes with this caring and loving therapy.

In the United States, it is not easy to find a well-trained Chinese massage doctor because there is no professional training school for this kind of therapy. Most massage schools teach regular massage, but only provide a little information on the oriental massage techniques.

Chinese massage works in the following ways:
- It works on the meridian system; it connects the upper and lower body, as well as the internal and external body.
- The strong and penetrating techniques stimulate Qi and blood circulation, which helps to break blockages, nourishes the whole body, and helps alleviate illness.

- It is related to nerve response: For example, acupuncture and massage can relieve pain due to endorphin and serotonin level changes in the brain, and changes in the potassium level between, inside, and outside cells.
- Chemical changes in the body (biochemical and neurochemical) occur due to stimulation of the energy passages.
- Changes in the autonomic nervous system.

In 2001, I took a group of Americans to China. We went to a rural mountain area, and hiked to the top of a mountain. While hiking, we had to carry backpacks so that our shoulders and backs hurt very much. Later that evening (after we returned to the hotel), I had a Chinese massage. The person doing the massage was trained as a TCM doctor with a massage specialty; he was only five-feet-three inches tall. During the massage, I felt the tremendous force from his hands. It was painful, I even screamed, but he did not hesitate and went on with his work, the kind smile never leaving his face. The next day, both my shoulders and my back felt much better. The Chinese massage might not be comfortable at the moment, but it certainly helps relieve your problems. Each time I take my students, patients, or other Americans to China, I want them to experience the unique healing benefits of Chinese massage. In the United States, Chinese massage needs to be modified with lighter manipulation because many people could not otherwise tolerate the massage's discomfort.

For example, putting pressure on the Yen Zhong point results in a cardiovascular response; this stimulates the sympathetic nervous system. Putting pressure on the Zhu San Li point results in a gastrointestinal response that stimulates the parasympathetic nerve system. Another point, called Yang Xi, results in an anti-parasympathetic nervous system response.

Self-Massage

Self-massage is another self-healing technique used by many Chinese people. It is a convenient and cost effective way to maintain good health. Many people use self-massage to help themselves and their family. It helps to boost the immune system, increase energy, and enhance the self-healing ability.

Picture yourself on an airplane. You begin to suffer from nausea or a headache, and you do not have any medication with you. If you know how to do self-massage, you can help yourself to relieve the discomfort. Otherwise, you would just have to suffer. If you see someone who has sunstroke, you could use massage techniques by pressing on the Ren Zhong point, which is located under your nose to save this person's life before the EMTs arrive.

Self-healing massage is an excellent tool for health maintenance. Most Chinese centenarians have always done some form of self-massage.

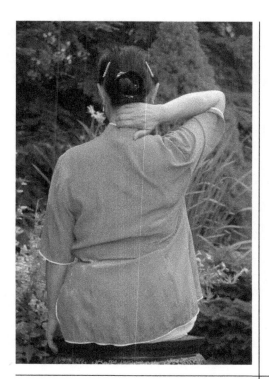

Relief of neck problems, stress, headache:

Put one hand across behind the neck, using fingers to massage the opposite side next to the muscle that is next to the cervical vertebrae. Use kneading, pressing methods. Start at bottom of scalp, gradually moving down to shoulder along the neck. Massage for two or three minutes, and then do opposite side.

Using forefinger and middle finger under scalp, 1.5 inches from middle line, using rotational pressure, massage this area for three minutes.

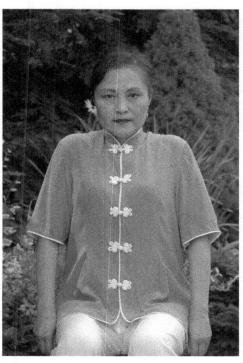

Circle both shoulders backwards 8 times, then circle both shoulders forward 8 times. Then hold both shoulders up for one deep inhale and make the shoulders tight, then drop the shoulders and relax the whole body while exhaling.

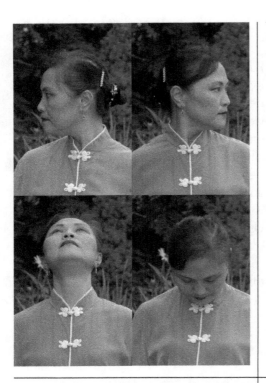

Neck exercise: slowly move the head in four directions, to the left, to the right, upward, and then downward.

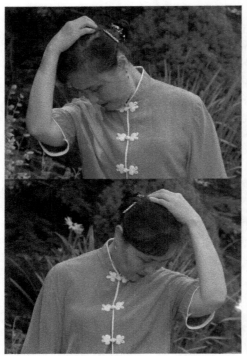

Hold head down with hand at 45-degree angle; press down with moderate pressure, and after one minute, switch to the other side. Now, with the head centered, hold head down with both hands and apply moderate pressure.

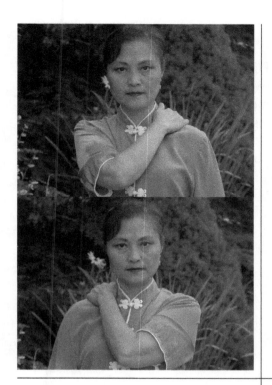

Using the opposite hand, massage shoulder muscles by crossing the arms across the chest.

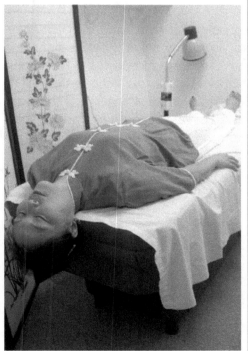

Lie down on a bed and move so your head hangs slightly from the edge of the bed. Let gravity pull down on your head providing natural neck traction. Do this for 1 minute.

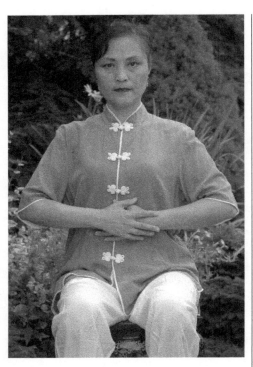

Gastrointestinal ailments, gassy stomach, indigestion:

Put hands over the upper stomach area (women, put right hand under left hand; men, put left hand under right hand); using rotational pressure, massage the upper stomach counterclockwise (to follow the colon pathway) for 2 or 3 minutes.

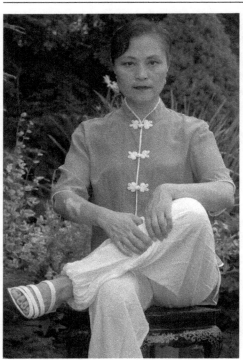

Leg point: Put right hand over left kneecap, your index finger is between the end of the kneecap and press the lateral tibia (shinbone) under the knee at the indent; the tip of the index finger is at the point you massage. Use pressing and kneading methods for 3 minutes. Then massage opposite leg, using same method to find the correct point on the other leg.

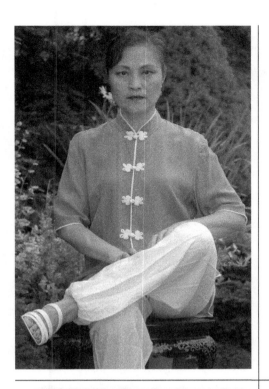

Massage the area under the knee joint at the inner part of the leg next to the shinbone; if you feel a little pain when you massage it, you will know if you have found the correct point.

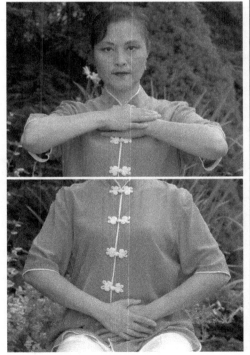

Put hands in the front of your chest. Men, put left hand under right hand; women, put right hand under left hand. Push down with pressure along the middle line of the front body 8 times; breathe out when you push down.

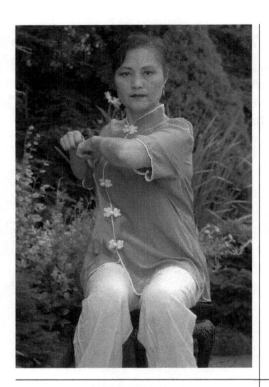

Alternately swing body (turn waist and torso, keep legs still) side-to-side 16 times.

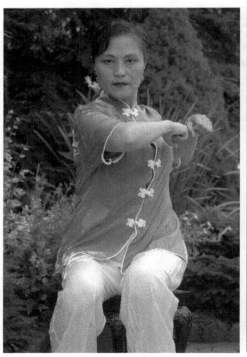

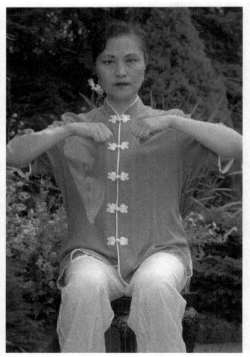

Other points used in self-healing massage

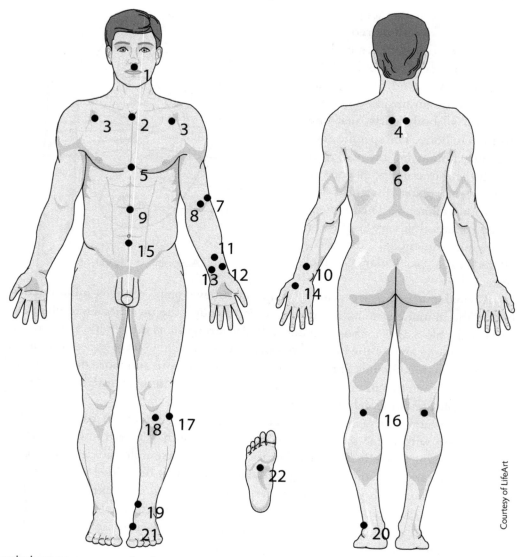

Courtesy of LifeArt

1. Lower back, emergency pressure point—fainting, unconsciousness
2. Cough, hoarseness, sore throat, immune system
3. Respiratory, chest cold, asthma, letting go/grief release
4. Neck, shoulder, back, bones
5. Pulmonary weakness, cough, chest pain, fluid buildup
6. Mid-thoracic tension, blood, skin, heart
7. Arm, skin
8. Respiratory
9. Upper abdomen
10. Hand, ear
11. Chest, heart, lungs, ribs
12. Neck
13. Emergency pressure point—anxiety heart palpitations

14. Face, head, eyes, ears, mouth, teeth
15. Lower abdomen, bladder, intestines, male/female organs, energy storehouse
16. Lower back, leg
17. Leg, knee, muscles, tendons
18. Upper abdomen, energizing point
19. Lower abdomen, large intestine, bladder
20. Foot, leg, upper back
21. Chest, ribs, depression, nervous system
22. Invigorating, awakens awareness of total body, promotes circulation of legs, back

NOTE: Points indicated on arm, hand, leg, or foot are located on either right or left arm, hand, leg, or foot.

Auricular Acupressure Therapy

Chinese auricular acupressure therapy is a time-honored treatment recorded in China's earliest medical books from over 2000 years ago. As noted earlier, your ear resembles an upside-down fetus, with all body parts, just like the human body. The specific acupressure points on the ear, just like the acupuncture points on the body, were treated for the relief of various ailments. This ancient healing method is very useful for balancing functional disorders related to a particular channel system.

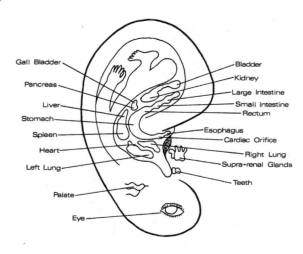

Acupoints in the ear.

Auricular acupressure therapy helps to relieve pain, reduces inflammation, boosts the immune system, increases energy through the meridians and channels, and breaks blockages in those channels. It also strengthens the function of and promotes harmony among the internal organs. Studies in China have shown that it can treat more than 200 kinds of functional disorders. As more and more doctors travel to China to learn this unique method so they can add it to their practice, more and more people are being helped by this therapy.

Chinese auricular acupressure therapy has no side effects. It can be used in combination with other therapies and treatments, both Western and Eastern. It helps reduce the side effects from other therapies. For example, side effects caused by chemotherapy, radiation, surgery, and medication can be helped with auricular acupressure therapy. It is also helpful in quitting smoking or drinking and in drug detoxification. Auricular therapy, combined with acupuncture, enhances healing. In addition to tongue and pulse diagnosis, Chinese doctors also use auricular therapy for diagnosis when there is an energy imbalance in the body.

During therapy, the practitioner puts a tiny herbal seed (sometimes a magnetic pellet is used) on certain points of the ear. Patients massage these points several times a day to stimulate them. Each point has close relationship to internal organs and body parts. When these points are stimulated, the internal organs and body parts are stimulated and the internal organ energy is activated.

Years ago, TCM practitioners used small needles to perform auricular acupuncture. Because there were side effects, nowadays most practitioners use herbs instead.

Chinese Herbal Medicine

China has vast resources for herbal medicines. The use of herbal medicine grew out of the Daoist idea that we came from nature; therefore, nature is the source for everything. The practice of herbal medicine developed before written language began, in a time when humans were still hunting and gathering food. People started to use different foods for relief of their ailments, gradually using different plants, then animal parts, then minerals, seashells, and so on.

The Chinese discovered medicinal herbs through thousands of years of trial and error. Some people died from using unknown poisonous plants or from overdoses of certain plants while others became very sick from the plants in the early days of medicinal herbal exploration. From the sickness and recovery after using the herbs, the Chinese gained a vast body of knowledge about herbal medicine, and passed it on, from generation to generation. Some people were cured by certain plants, and others felt more energetic after taking the plants. Still other people felt less pain after using the plants and herbs. After many years trying and testing, the Chinese developed a complete medical herbal system for health care, disease prevention, and longevity.

Chinese herbal medicine is the most popular treatment used in TCM practices in China. Most Chinese people use Chinese herbal medicine, which is much more popular than acupuncture. Chinese herbal medicine has its own unique way, which is completely different from Western herbal medicine, in that it rarely uses a single herb for healing. The herbs are prescribed by Chinese doctors or acupuncturists, in much the same way Western doctors prescribe pharmaceutical medication to their patients—mostly a single drug or two. In Chinese prescriptions, some herbal prescriptions have 4 different herbs; others contain 10 different herbs; while others even contain 20 different herbs. To make up a prescription, the TCM doctor carefully blends a number of herbs, which have specific functions to balance specific organs or other disharmonies. Each herb has its own task: reducing inflammation; speeding up metabolism; enhancing energy; promoting blood circulation; and so on. Chinese herbalists prescribe herbs to strengthen several organs to balance the energy. Since every human body is different, Chinese doctors treat patients with individualized prescriptions, even if two people have the same symptoms. For instance, two people suffering from bronchitis might receive a different herbal prescription; one can be for relief of a "cold-caused" bronchitis; the other can be for relief of a "heat-caused" bronchitis.

Textbooks on herbal medicine in TCM describe formulations that are made from the roots, stems, bark, leaves, seeds, or flowers of many plants, as well as some minerals and animal parts. These days, because the world is concerned about animal rights and endangered species, animal products are used much less in herbal treatments, and eventually they will not be used at all.

The herbs are usually decocted into a soup, which must be cooked twice. These herbs do not taste as good as herbs we use for cooking; in fact, you really have to hold your nose when you drink this soup! Usually, whole plant herbs are taken in the form of a "recipe" called a TCM herbal prescription. Some herbs come in ready-prepared pills or powders, called patent herbal remedies. The pill form is less effective than real/whole herb plants that require cooking, but they can still be effective and, of course, the pill form is much more convenient than cooked herbs.

There are many different herb categories: tonic and detoxifying herbs, herbs that promote Qi and blood circulation or dispel cold, dampness, and heat, induce elimination, or reduce elimination by inducing or reducing sweating; combat infection, reduce coughing, dispel mucus, stop bleeding, activate blood, induce water elimination, improve digestive functions, or improve skin problems; calm the mind, help sleeping; and much more.

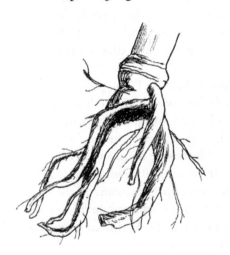

Dang Gui, a blood tonic.

Chinese herbal medicine has had a long history of treating mental illness. Zhang Zhong Jin (150-219), a famous TCM doctor in Chinese medical history (described earlier in this book), recorded techniques treating all types of mental illness with various herbal prescriptions, thus indicating that herbal medicine has been effective in treating mental illness for many centuries, and that mental illness responds to natural treatments. Chinese herbal medicine treatments for mental illness are totally individualized. Two people who have depression, for example, can have two very different herbal prescriptions. It all depends on which organ has blockage, stagnation, or disharmony. The experienced TCM doctor can prescribe a very effective preparation.

Chinese herbal medicine also has a long history of use in treating cancer. Not only do some herbal medicines have an anticancer effect, but many herbs also enhance the immune function, an important factor in cancer healing. Through harmonized organ energy, the cancer patients heal faster and the tumor gradually reduces in size and hardness, thereby removing the blockage to body parts.

In fact, if used appropriately, Chinese herbal medicine can treat almost everything. Herbs can be harmful if they are not used correctly. An overdose or wrong combination of herbs can cause problems. Some herbs with low toxicity can be very effective for certain diseases. Therefore, one must follow the instruction of a qualified practitioner to avoid side effects. For children and seniors, practitioners must be more careful; for them the dosage should be much less. In Western medicine, there are also some drugs that are toxic, but still helpful for relief of certain conditions.

Seeking the Right Medical Care

When a person is ill, most times he or she calls the doctor right way, while minor ailments are usually ignored. Oftentimes, the minor ailment can be healed; but in other cases, the minor problem can be a sign of major illness. For this reason, one should not ignore small physical problems. On the other hand, a small problem can be fixed easily, while the larger problems are more difficult to fix and require a longer period of time to treat. In most cases, your doctor is able to help you when your self-healing ability is strong. If your problem is more than the doctor can handle, you should search for other avenues to treatment. Here are suggestions that might help your healing journey.

- **For acute illness**, the Western doctor's prescription can be helpful for relieving symptoms quickly. However, TCM care is also a good choice because it has no side effects, unless the condition is life threatening. The choice of treatment is yours, but the decision can be limited due to

I had a patient who became sick after eating a sandwich at a company's conference; the lunch was catered by a Vietnamese restaurant. Two days later, she was very sick with vomiting, diarrhea, and abdominal pain. She went to the emergency room for IV fluids and antibiotics, but nothing seemed to help. The diarrhea and abdominal pain continued, with occasional vomiting. Her appetite was poor and she lost weight. She went to see a doctor many times and had many tests done. Finally, the doctor found out that she had an amoeba, which is rare in the United States but common in Asian countries. Since it was rare, not much attention was paid to this type of illness, and not many drugs were available for this rare condition. She finally came to me for help. After knowing what it was, I decided to use herbs to treat her. I contacted a friend, a classmate in medical school in China and now a specialist in infectious diseases. My friend had not seen this condition either because it is also rare in China. She suggested some medication that was not available in the United States. I looked in many TCM books, and finally found the herbal prescription for amoeba. I gave my patient a three-week supply of these herbs. Her symptoms started getting better after the first week, and was much better by the end of the third week. By the fourth week, she was completely well. In this particular case, when Western medicine could not help her, TCM proved to be beneficial. In her prescription, I included anti-parasite herbs (which are slightly toxic), and herbs to nourish the bowels, reduce diarrhea, enhance energy, as well as blood tonics. This prescription balanced her body and immune system, leading her to complete healing. Cases like this are similar to chemotherapy, in which the toxic medication helps to kill the cancer cells. In order to heal the body, we sometimes need the heavy-duty, toxic medicine, or herbs to help to fight disease.

insurance issues. In China, since insurance covers both kinds of treatment, it does not matter if an illness is acute or chronic; some people only use TCM care, while others only use conventional medicine.

- **For chronic illness**, it is better to go to a TCM doctor. Many people do not have enough knowledge to seek out TCM and their frustration only makes their illness worse. Although taking prescription drugs can help relieve symptoms, taking them too long can impair your organ energy system, or you might develop other problems more dangerous than your current condition. Chinese medicine can help you not only get rid of the symptoms, but also correct the root cause of the problem and enhance your self-healing ability. Due to these benefits, TCM has excellent results in treating chronic ailments than Western medicine, and it is worthwhile to have TCM care in these instances.

- **For minor complaints**, you should start an exercise plan. Regular walking, practicing Qigong and Taiji will give you a balanced workout. These exercises promote Qi circulation and indirectly promote blood circulation, which helps balance internal organ energy. In this way, your minor symptoms gradually recede. You might surprise yourself as to how well you feel after practicing Qigong and Taiji for a while.

- **If you have an injury without a fracture**, such as soft tissue injury on your back due to incorrect posture or back sprain, Chinese herbal medicine and acupuncture are the best treatment. Without acupuncture treatments, your back sprain can last weeks or months, even years. With acupuncture treatment, you can go back to work within one week with only minimal symptoms or discomfort. Many herbal remedies exist for muscle contusions that help muscle tissue heal faster. For instance, I had experiences with muscle pain when I was in college. Like a miracle, the herbal medicine quickly worked to heal the injury.

- **If you have low energy**, try Chinese medicine. Western medicine looks into the structural elements of the problem. Without observable structural abnormalities, Western medicine may not always treat low energy effectively. You should get acupuncture treatment for a tune up. Low energy has many different causes, including virus, yeast, or bacterial infections; hormone imbalance, high stress, family disharmony, tumors, mental or other chronic illnesses. Viral infections do not respond to antibiotics because the virus resides in the cells and using chemicals to kill the virus also kills the host cells. Your immune system can keep viruses quiet in the body for many years, so they do not cause any visible problems. TCM enhances the immune system, which is why people who have had regular TCM care have fewer infections. TCM care improves energy and smooths the meridian pathways, thus making you feel better. You would be surprised what TCM can do for you. Despite my training as a Western medical doctor in China, even I was surprised by how much TCM can make people feel better. Some patients who had special (rare) illnesses, which I initially thought TCM could not help, improved after TCM treatments. During my own practice of TCM, I have seen many astonishing results, even when I did not believe the patients would get better at first. TCM is the first step of natural healing.

- **Functional problems:** If you have not been feeling well for a long time and your doctor cannot find anything wrong because the tests do not help identify any specific problem, you have a functional problem rather than anatomical or structural problem. Your Chinese doctor might tell you that your organ energy is not working together. Your internal balance is lost, and you need a tune up treatment to restore the balance.

- **If your body cannot tolerate the side effects of a medication** you are taking, you should look into Chinese and other alternative medicines. If used under professional care, Chinese medicine has no side effects.

- **For chronic muscle problems**, Chinese massage is the first choice; it can be used in combination with acupuncture for better results.

- **For children**, TCM treatments provide excellent results. If a child were afraid of acupuncture, Chinese massage would be the first choice of treatment. Other alternative therapies might also help. Children heal faster than adults do.

- **For infections**, you need to go to a Western doctor to get antibiotics. Herbal medicine can treat infection, but it is too mild for certain infections. There are strong herbs the TCM doctor could prescribe, but children would not like the unpleasant taste.

- **For mild mental ailments**, such as anxiety, depression, or panic attacks, you should do both Western and Eastern exercises. If the duration of the mental ailment is too long, or if the condition is too severe, you will probably need medication from your doctor. If you do not want to take the medication over the long term, talk to a doctor who might help you slowly discontinue use of the medication. In any case, it is better to get TCM treatment at the same time.

- **For addiction**, Chinese medicine is a good choice, but only if you really want to quit. There are support groups available, and they are a good way to get help; but when combined with TCM treatment, you will become balanced at the same time you are treating the addiction.

- **For premenstrual syndrome (PMS)**, Chinese medicine does a wonderful job. It not only relieves the symptoms but also delays the aging process.

In China, I rarely saw PMS during my practice as an obstetrician/gynecologist, and the rate of breast cancer was low, too.

- **For stomach problems**, Chinese herbal medicine should be your first choice. In addition to relieving symptoms, the herbs improve stomach energy. Once your stomach energy improves, other organs also improve because stomach energy supports other organ energies. Because they know how to use herbs effectively, many Chinese people take herbs immediately when they have stomach and intestine problems.

- **For neuromuscular problems**, you should get treatment with acupuncture before starting to take medication. In many cases, acupuncture can relieve the pain. In China, these are the most common problems that are treated with acupuncture. If the acupuncture treatments do not help, you then take medication or other therapies prescribed by your primary care doctor.

- **For shingles**, definitely go to an acupuncturist because it works beautifully to relieve the pain.

You should always correct small ailments to avoid bigger problems. Using TCM care can prevent many devastating problems in the future. Prevention is the focus of TCM practice.

Regarding herbal tonics, one has to be careful using them. Herbal tonics are generally good for the body for people who need them, but the results can vary from person to person. Your TCM doctor should help you learn what your body's physical constitution is, and what you are treating with the herb. Using an herb for the wrong physical constitution can cause adverse effects. For instance, if a patient who has hypertension takes ginseng (Ren Shen, also called Gin Shen) for a long time, the blood pressure may elevate. In this case, too much Yang causes a traffic jam, of sorts. On the other hand, if you take a Yin tonic for Yin-type body constitution (cold-type body), your symptoms would not be better because too much Yin causes depletion of Yang energy. If you have pain that is caused by stagnation of blood (from an old or new injury), you should use herbs that promote blood and Qi circulation. Because the Qi drives the blood, we often use both types of herbs at the same time.

Around 1998, there was a report about a person who died from taking herbal medicine. A big controversy about Chinese herbal medicine followed that led to many Chinese herbs being removed from the market. Some of them were very useful in healing even though they were mildly toxic (much less toxic than chemotherapy). Many doctors suggested patients not take Chinese herbs. However, the reason the person died from taking herbs was that he took too much and for far too long without TCM professional advice.

Part II

Healing and Prevention

Chapter 2

Food Healing in Chinese Medicine

The Importance of Food Healing

Food and health have a very close relationship. Many illnesses can be caused by consuming the wrong foods, too much food, or unhealthy eating habits. Bad eating habits can lead to heart disease, hypertension, high cholesterol, diabetes, obesity, liver disease, gastrointestinal disease, asthma, insomnia, and many other illnesses. Based on testimonials from Chinese doctors, the rates of heart disease, diabetes, and hypertension were much lower in China during the 1960s and 1970s than they are now. New data from the *Boston Globe* in 2003 reported that 112 million Chinese have cholesterol between 200 and 239. Another 42 million have cholesterol levels above 240 and are at especially high risk of heart attack. A total of 102 million Americans have cholesterol levels over 200. An estimated 26 million Chinese have diabetes compared to 16 million in the U.S. It is estimated that 30 percent of adults have some degree of hypertension; furthermore, obesity in children is also increasing. I believe that one reason these health conditions are changing is diet. The Chinese diet has changed significantly in the past 20 years. These days, in China, you can find many Western-style, fast-food restaurants that are just as popular as in the U.S. Due to their fast-paced and busy lifestyles, more and more people eat fast food daily; more and more people eat restaurant food, rather than home cooking. Despite the change in lifestyle, many Chinese still do their daily exercise, which has certainly reduced many other illnesses.

There is a much higher rate of weight problems in China now than before, especially in children. Many young people

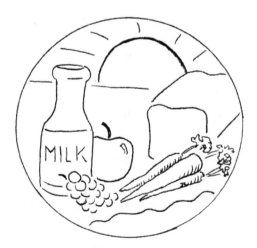

Food Healing

think they do not need to watch their diet because they are healthy now, which is faulty reasoning that can lead to a potentially unhealthy future. Weight problems in childhood most likely will cause weight problems in adulthood.

"Obesity is related more to what people eat then how much. Adjusted for height, the Chinese consume 20 percent more calories than Americans do. But Americans are 25 percent fatter. The main dietary differences are fat and starch. The Chinese eat only a third the amount of fat Americans do, while eating twice the starch. The body readily stores fat, but expends a large proportion of the carbohydrates consumed as heat. Some of the difference may be attributable to exercise…." (From the *New York Times*, May 8, 1990).

Our Chinese ancestors knew the importance of the relationship between food, weight, and disease. In the Tang Dynasty, the famous Dr. Sun Si-Miao said that when a person is sick, the doctor should first regulate the patient's diet and lifestyle. In most cases, these changes alone are enough to effect a cure over time. He added that only if changes in diet and lifestyle are not enough should the doctor administer other interventions, such as herbal medicine and acupuncture.

Patients coming for TCM treatment or therapies still need to change their diet and lifestyle for the TCM treatment to be more effective. During many years of clinical experience, I have seen many cases in which the difference in the success of treatments depends on whether or not the diet was changed. Some patients improved just from changing the food they consumed; others periodically got sick even with many acupuncture visits. Part of the reason was that they were not willing to change their diet and lifestyle.

Foods and Diets Causing Blockage and Imbalance

Diet is very important in our lives. With correct diet, we may enjoy life to the fullest. Food and diet can cause blockages in our body; these blockages can result from any of 9 categories of excesses:

- Too much food
- Too many calories
- Too much meat
- Too much dairy
- Too many sweets
- Too much cold food and cold drinks
- Too much "eat out" food
- Too much spicy food
- Too much fast food or preserved food

Healing and Digestion

In Chinese healing, the digestive function is one of the most important issues because it affects healing for the whole body. If the digestive system goes wrong, eventually something will go wrong in the other organs. This is especially true for cancer patients; if the patients still have good digestive function, their prognosis improves.

Maintaining good stomach energy is especially important for women. Good stomach function helps prevent breast cancer. In the body meridian system, the Stomach Meridian goes through the breast. If the Stomach Meridian is blocked, it might cause a blockage on the breast, which could be a pre-cancer area. If we look at breast cancer patients' medical histories, not including genetic factors, we find many of them in their lifetime had some kind of problem in their stomach function. Some people had stomach problems when they were young, others in middle age, and still others had just recently experienced stomach problems. Of course, there are other causes of breast cancer such as genetic factors and blockages in certain energy paths.

Preserving stomach energy is a large part of preserving one's daily energy level, too. Just recall your daily life: Do you feel tired after eating a good-size lunch? What do you feel if you do not eat big meals at lunchtime? These questions can be your homework to find out about your energy level.

Any stomach discomfort or problem should not be ignored, but should be corrected before the condition turns into a long-term problem.

I had one patient who told me she would like to lose weight. She had been eating late dinners for many years and was unwilling to change. The day she told me she could not change was when I knew it was going to be difficult for her to lose the extra weight. At the end of her treatments, the results were poor. There are many successful cases of treating weight problems with acupuncture and herbs; but most of these patients also changed their diet. Their weight dropped between 5 to 20 pounds thus indicating that the kinds of foods they ate played a very important role in weight control. Changing diet involves changing one's eating habits and lifestyle.

Guidelines to Chinese Food Healing

The Chinese use of food for healing has a long history. Today it is still popular in China due to its great value in preventing disease and its contribution to longevity. Some methods of food healing the Chinese use are similar to Western food curative principles. For instance, the food we use for treating night blindness has a high vitamin A content. For goiters, the food used for healing would be seaweed or sea vegetable, which contains high amounts of iodine. For anemia, the foods containing high amounts of iron would be used. The principle is that you eat what you lack in the body.

Chinese food healing is different from Western nutrition, which considers how much protein, carbohydrate, vitamins, minerals, and fat are being taken in. Chinese food healing uses food to balance the body's energy makes use of a healthy and balanced diet, recommends that patients eat the right food to assist healing, and naturally maintains optimum body weight. Take tofu (bean curd, made from soybean) for example. The Westerner pays attention to what is in the tofu, its nutritional value, and how it is made; Chinese food healing, on the other hand, considers not only tofu's nutritional value, but also uses the cooling feature of tofu to balance the body's energy.

A man suffering from advanced cancer came to me with very poor energy. His stomach energy was very poor, too. I knew that he had end-stage cancer and it was too late to save his life. I tried to restore his organs' energy, especially stomach energy, along with treatment to boost his immune function. In two weeks, he was feeling much better. His digestive function, energy, attitude, and sleeping improved, and his pain lessened, etc. When he went back for chemotherapy, he did not have the time and strength to continue the TCM treatment. As a result, he started to lose his appetite, and then lost his daily energy level; he got pneumonia soon after. When he came back to our clinic after several weeks, I knew it was too late, and shortly afterward, he passed away.

Requires learning and understanding: Food healing requires learning, understanding, and discipline for it to be consistent. A healthy mind gives you better results, which is what you want. This means your mind is the most important element in food healing. Many people do not have patience; they are looking for immediate results or a quick cure. This impediment could prevent people from reaching their goal or seeing results. Food healing needs time to be effective, from several weeks to a lifetime. For instance, if you are allergic to a specific food, you might have to avoid this food throughout your entire lifetime. If you have been eating the wrong foods for many years and have physical problems that might be caused by the foods you consume, you might need to eat different foods for a while before seeing changes in your physical condition. If you have a Yang-type physical constitution, which appears to have hot or warm symptoms more often, you should eat more Yin-type food, which has cooling features in order to balance your body. If you continue to eat more Yang-type food, you can accumulate too much Yang energy in the body, leading to an imbalance of the organ system that causes the symptoms, or makes them worse. You may develop some other physical problem. As we discussed before, either too much Yin or Yang can cause problems.

Need to be flexible: Food healing sometimes requires that an individual be more flexible. Sometimes the body constitution changes temporarily and you need to pay attention to the present status of your body. For instance, you may have a Yang-type body constitution, but you get a cold, which means your present body constitution has become Yin for this time. You need to include more Yang-type food (such as ginger soup) in your diet temporarily to deal with the cold. Later, when the cold is better, your body might change back to its original Yang-type body. You then eat more Yin-types of food to balance your body's constitution. If your body type changes to normal, neither Yin- nor Yang-type, you then eat whatever you enjoy and eat a variety of foods. For some people, the body might not change back to its original type after the illness. The bottom line is to pay attention to your present body type.

Mind plays important role: Your mind is the most important element in food healing. It all depends on how you think, how you want to think, how determined you are, what your goal is, and how you can reach your goal. For some people who have strong minds and are determined, if they want to lose 30 pounds in three months, they would do anything to achieve this. For many people, it could be a very difficult thing to do.

Food healing cannot substitute for medicine: Food healing cannot substitute for medicine; rather, it is complementary to medical treatments. Some people tend to do things to the extreme; others rely too much on medication; and still others strongly believe food is the only way. None of these is correct. Eating the right food is important in maintaining a good daily energy level and an appropriate weight. Regarding healing, eating the right food should be done in conjunction with other therapies, either Western or Eastern medicine. With serious medical ailments, you need to see your doctor for medical assistance.

Is food the energy source, yes or no?: Many people think food is the energy source. Yes, if the foods you eat are digested and absorbed appropriately; no, if the foods you eat are not digested and absorbed appropriately. Yes, if you eat the appropriate amount and no, if you do not eat the appropriate amount. If you have spleen energy deficiency, which is correlated to digestive function, no matter how well you eat you will still be fatigued. Many people often think the more food you eat the more energy you will have. The fact is, the more you eat, the less energy you will have, unless your job requires heavy physical labor, in which case you do need more food for energy. The Chinese diet concept is very different from the Western diet concept. Since each individual is different, each should try to change food habits to determine his or her own ideal, balanced diet.

In summary, food healing involves:
1. Using food to balance the body's energy.
2. A healthy and balanced diet.
3. Eating the right foods to assist healing.
4. Maintaining optimum weight, naturally.

Food Balance

It is common sense that you would have hot soup in the wintertime and ice cream during the summer. Most of the time, you know how to balance food. If you feel cold, you eat or drink warm foods; if you feel hot, you eat or drink cold foods. Food healing, however, is more complicated because the body is a complicated system and things do not always work the way we think they should. If a person gets a cold, he might feel a chill, but at the same time may have a fever; in this case, food healing can be confusing. Should the person use hot food to balance cold, or should cold food be used to balance the fever?

Food has energy just as humans do. The energy of food refers to its capacity to generate sensation – either hot or cold – in the human body. For example, eating food with a hot energy will give us a hot sensation; we feel warm as long as the food is still in our system. Conversely, eating food with cold energy will give us a cold sensation.

Hot or cold energy in food does not necessarily refer to the present state of the food. For example, green tea has cold energy, even though it is served hot; it still is considered a cooling beverage. Shortly after the tea enters your body, its heat (a temporary phenomenon) will be lost, and as it begins to generate cold energy, your body begins to cool off. That is why in the hot summer, you like to drink a bottle of iced tea to cool you off. Chinese people eat many mung beans in the summer such as mung bean porridge, because mung beans have protein and carbohydrates, and it can also cool you. Even though you eat cold, spicy red pepper, you will still feel hot after, because the red hot pepper generates heat.

For balancing the body energy, herbs are more effective than food (because herbs last longer) while food is more effective than water.

Food Used to Assist Healing

If you have arthritis, the symptoms are always worse in the cold and damp weather, because most arthritis is caused by excessive coldness and dampness. You will feel better by eating warm or hot food on a regular basis, in the same way that you feel better after using a hot pack over an arthritic area. Scientists in the United States, who researched the use of hot pepper for relief from arthritis pain, found out that applying hot pepper juice externally helped to reduce pain and chronic inflammation. I am not sure if they really understood the concepts of cold energy and hot energy, but this study coincides with TCM principles. Their theory is that capsaicin is the main chemical in hot pepper that relieves arthritis pain.

If you have skin problems, the symptom is worsened when you are exposed to heat, because most skin problems are caused by excessive heat. The symptoms would be relieved by eating cold or cool foods on a regular basis. If you continue to eat foods with hot energy, your symptoms will worsen.

Food Has Energy

Foods have energy just as everything else has energy. Understanding food energy can help us to eat a better diet and obtain better health. For example, leafy vegetables are cold, root vegetables are warm.

- **Food with cold energy:** bamboo shoots, banana, bitter gourd, clam, clamshell, crab, grapefruit, kelp, lettuce, lotus plumules, muskmelon, persimmon, salt, sea grass, seaweed, star fruit, sugarcane, water chestnut, watermelon.

- **Food with slightly cold energy:** hops, tomatoes.

- **Food with cooling energy:** apple, barley, bean curd, egg white, cucumber, eggplant, lettuce, lily flower, mandarin orange, mango, marjoram, mung bean, oyster shell, pear, peppermint, radish, sesame oil, spinach, strawberry, tangerine, wheat.

- **Food with hot energy:** black pepper, cinnamon bark, cottonseed, ginger, green pepper, red pepper, soybean oil, white pepper.

- **Food with neutral energy:** apricot, beef, black fungus, black sesame seeds, black soybean, Chinese cabbage, carrot, celery, egg yolk, corn, corn silk, crab apple, duck, fig, grape, honey, kidney bean, milk, olive, oyster, peanuts, pineapple, plum, pork, potato, pumpkin, radish leaf, string bean, sunflower seeds, sweet potato, white sugar, yellow soybean.

- **Food with warm energy:** brown sugar, cherry, chestnut, chicken, chive, cinnamon stick, clove, coconut, coffee, date, fennel, garlic, fresh ginger, ginseng (Ren Shen), green onion, ham, leaf mustard, leek, nutmeg, peach, raspberry, rosemary, shrimp, squash, basil, vinegar, wine, walnut.

> I had a patient who had bad psoriasis, and one day she told me her skin problem was worse. I asked her if she drank liquor the previous evening, and she said yes, that she went out with friends and had several drinks. I explained to her that liquor has hot energy, and that the skin problem is due to too much heat (Yang) in the body. This excessive Yang energy in the body caused her skin problem to become worse. I suggested that she needed to avoid liquor. After she stopped drinking it, her skin improved. I also suggested that she should drink more green tea to balance her body energy. Food balancing the body energy requires an understanding of what food energy and body constitution are all about.

Plants that take longer to grow are more warming than those that grow quickly. Raw food is more cooling than cooked food. Deep fried food is more warming. Food eaten cold is more cooling. Regarding food color, the green, purple, blue, or white foods are usually more cooling than red, orange, or yellow foods. Regarding cooking methods, foods that need longer cooking times, higher temperature or higher pressure are more warming; whereas, foods that require less time to cook are more cooling. Chemically fertilized plants are more cooling than organic plants.

Physical Constitutions in the Human Body

There are six types of physical constitutions: hot, cold, dry, damp, deficient, excessive.

In a healthy person, the body's constitution should be neutral; even with a specific type of body constitution, there should be no symptoms. If the body constitution is dominant, and causes symptoms that affect our daily life, it is a sign of imbalance that needs to be corrected.

Hot physical constitution: Feels hot, dislikes heat, tongue red with yellow coating, facial skin mostly red or hot, urine appears yellow, stool is hard, sometimes has nose bleeds or canker sores sweats more than normal or has night sweats, always likes to drink ice-cold water (even in winter), wears less clothes, does not like summer.

Cold physical constitution: Feels cold, even in a room with a temperature that other people consider comfortable; likes to drink warm or room temperature water; the tongue appears white with a thin and white coating. Skin is pale or cold, urine appears light in color or has no color, stool often loose; rarely sweats.

Dry physical constitution: Often thirsty; nose, lips, throat, skin are all dry; dry cough, frequently constipated, tends to be skinny.

Damp physical constitution: Sometimes it can be difficult to identify. You feel heavy, tired, tongue appears glossy and greasy; gains weight easily, often has water retention, often overweight, weak, low energy; women often have PMS symptoms.

Deficient physical constitution (can be mixed with hot, cold, damp, or dry body constitutions): Feels weak, low energy, low spirit, pale complexion, frequently feels tired, perspires excessively, palpitation or shortness of breath, tongue appears clear without coating. Often thin. Often suffers from prolapsed organs due to lack of energy to support the internal organs.

Excessive physical constitution (can be mixed with hot, cold, damp or dry body constitutions): Strong and energetic, high spirited, speaks in high-pitched voice, easily irritated, often has reddish complexion, may have constipation, poor sleep patterns, attention-deficient disorder, mania, hypertension, or heart disease.

Determining the body's constitution can be complicated. People often have mixed physical constitutions, such as cold and dry, damp and hot, cold and deficient, or some other combination. Sometimes the body's internal and external constitutions can be completely opposite, such as internal hot and external cold, or internal cold and external hot. Only an experienced TCM practitioner will be able to identify the constitution correctly.

Balanced Diets

Each individual has a different physical constitution and requires a different diet to become balanced. We should follow these principles.

Just as I would like to help my friend get better from her long lasting skin problem, I am writing this book partly to help you understand that food can help you if you are willing to change your diet.

Correction Strategies for Imbalances

1. If you have cold-type physical constitution (Yin): You should eat food with warm or hot energy (sweet and pungent). You should try to avoid food with cold energy, such as bitter foods. Coffee has hot energy; it is good for a cold-type body constitution (but drink it in moderation). Green tea has cold energy, so it is not appropriate to drink in excess. Since green tea has many other benefits to our body, we drink it for those benefits, and use it with some other warming food to balance our body. If you catch a cold, ginger soup will make you feel better, because ginger has warming features. If you have a cold stomach, black pepper can help you, because black pepper is warm to our stomach. Some Chinese herbs like Yang tonics can be used in extreme cases, such as ginseng (Ren Shen), Astragalus (Huang Qi), licorice (Gan Cao), cinnamon bark (Rou Gui), aconite (Fu Zi), Epimedium (Yin Yang Huo), Psoralea (Bu Gu Zi), Polygonatum (Huang Jing), Dioscorea (Shan Yao). If you want to use herbs, you should consult a qualified TCM practitioner thus helping you avoid side effects and obtain better results.

2. If you have a hot-type physical constitution (Yang): You should eat more food with cold or cool energy. Green tea has cold energy; it is good for balancing a hot-type body, especially in the summer (you do not have to drink hot green tea in the summer). You should eat less meat, and eat more vegetables; you should avoid alcohol, smoking, coffee, and fried food. This is part of maintaining balance

One of my friends had a bad rash on her hands and feet all her life. For a long time, I had been asking her to change her diet and do some kind of self-care. She did not want to change her diet and did not do the self-care. The rashes on her hands and feet never improved. There might be temporary relief for a very short time, and then the rash would return. In Chinese medicine, any kind of skin rash indicates that the body lost its Yin-Yang balance. Chinese doctors always look for external signs to identify internal imbalances. They then treat the internal organ and bring balance so that the external rash disappears. My friend's rash on both her hands and feet indicates that she has accumulated heat toxins in her body. The internal body has heat toxins, but they appear on the surface of the body: sometimes on the torso, sometimes on the back, sometimes on the hands or feet, or sometimes on the face. My friend's diet is very Yang and she has a stressful job, factors that cause her skin problem and makes it hard to heal. Her case may be a little too advanced for food therapy alone. Just changing her diet is not enough; she needed a combination of changing her diet and Chinese herbal medicine applied both internally and externally, as well as acupuncture to help her reduce her stress.

for your body type. For chronic constipation from excessive heat in the body, you should eat more leafy vegetables, which have cold energy. If you consume food with hot energy, such as hot pepper or alcohol, any symptoms you might become worse; you might also develop hemorrhoids. Drinking warm milk every morning or other warm liquids with honey can help you relieve constipation. Eating bananas can also help relieve constipation. If you have hives, eating mung bean soup can relieve the symptoms because mung bean has cold energy. For people who have a hot-type body constitution, liquor can cause such symptoms as skin rash, headache, stomach problems, nose bleeding, and constipation due to too much Yang accumulated in the body. Each individual can develop different symptoms. Liquor can also cause symptoms to worsen. For example, you might have heard about people saying that their skin rash is always worse after drinking alcohol.

In Chinese medicine, eating food with cold energy can help to relieve alcohol overdose. For example, in China, people often give the person who has overdosed on alcohol strong green tea to neutralize the alcohol in the body.

3. If you have a dry-type physical constitution (Yang): You should eat more food that lubricates dryness like honey, drink more liquids, eat more fruits and vegetables, and avoid dry food, such as nuts and chips. In the U.S., the dry-body constitution is uncommon; the damp body constitution is more common. The dry-type body constitution is more common in men than in women.

4. If you have a damp-type physical constitution (Yin): This is the type of body that gains weight easily. It can be explained by problems with water retention or water metabolism. The damp-type body constitution is more common in women than in men, especially in the U.S. Men can also have this kind of body constitution. In Western medicine, some medical practitioners suggest patients use diuretics to drain water (excess water in certain areas of the body) from the body. This method can cause both imbalance of electrolytes in the body and more imbalance of water metabolism.

In TCM, the strategy for balancing the damp constitution includes naturally promoting urination (from certain foods), increasing perspiration (from exercise), and eating aromatic foods to dry the body. Eating foods that can promote water passage, such as cucumber, watermelon, winter melon, small red beans (adzuki), corn, and corn silk can help you lose water. Eating aromatic or spicy foods will help you dry the organs. Certain bean products can help absorb the water (e.g., broad beans, hyacinth beans). You should also avoid food that produces more fluid, such as eating less salt and dairy. Dairy products cause excessive production of mucus that leads to imbalances in water metabolism. In the United States, many people consume too many dairy products; this is part of the reason that there are many cases of chronic fatigue syndrome, overweight, and PMS.

Regular exercise that induces sweating is an important way to lose body water. I have observed that many people do not like to be sweaty. I understand that sweating is not comfortable, but there are benefits. From the Yin-Yang philosophy, we know there are two sides to everything—the good side, and the bad side. The bad side of sweating is discomfort and odor; but the good side of sweating is that you burn calories, lose water and, therefore, lose weight, improve circulation, and feel more energetic. Obviously, there are more benefits in healthy sweat that is produced from exercise, which is considered the normal way of sweating. Some people sweat without a good amount of exercise or any other reason. This is not normal, indicating an imbalance of Yin-Yang. Too much Yang in the body or not enough Yin can cause abnormal sweating. In this case, you need to see a TCM practitioner. In general, the more you can make yourself sweat, the more water you can lose. You should do more cardio workouts, power walking, or aerobic exercises to perspire more. This activity will help you to lose more water and speed up your metabolism. Practicing Qigong and Taiji exercises can improve the energy and blood circulation, which can also improve whole body metabolism, helping you to lose water indirectly. Many people who have a damp-type body also have low energy, which discourages them from exercising. If this is your case, you need to push yourself to start, start with a mild form of exercise. Once you feel better, you will be encouraged and do even more.

People who have the damp-physical constitution need to watch their diet throughout their lives, unless the body type changes (body constitution could change in some people). If the body is too damp and has already caused problems that affect your life, you should see a TCM practitioner for acupuncture treatments. You can also take some Chinese herbs, such as Poria (Fu Ling), Atractylodes (Bai Zu), Coix seeds (Yi Yi Ren), small red beans (adzuki), etc. There are many patent Chinese herbs that can help to promote water metabolism, such as Jian Pi Wan, Shen Ling Bai Shu Shan, etc. Your practitioner can prescribe these for you.

5. If you have a deficient type physical constitution (Yin): Most people with this deficiency type have weak organ energy. It needs more than just eating the right foods to be corrected. The TCM doctor can increase your energy using many different methods such as acupuncture or Chinese herbs. Herbal tonics such as ginseng (Ren Shen), Astragalus (Huang Qi), and licorice (Gan Cao) are safe to take if you cannot find a good practitioner. You should eat foods that provide energy, such as yams, Mexican yams, and other root vegetables, or red dates. Yams contain protein, carbohydrates, calcium, and vitamins, and can strengthen your kidneys. People with deficient body types need to practice Taiji and Qigong, which can strengthen energy and blood circulation. They also need to practice Chinese exercise throughout their lifetime.

6. If you have an excessive type physical constitution (Yang): You should avoid tonics and consume fewer stimulants. People who have hypertension should not take ginseng and other Yang tonics, which might make the blood pressure higher. Eat more vegetables and fruit, and eat more food with cooling energy. Eat less meat, sugar, and dairy. For this kind of body type, any food that is too heavy will worsen the symptoms.

Organs' balanced diet: Eating a variety of foods is important, because doing so balances all organs. Picky eaters usually have some sort of imbalance in their organ system; some organ might be too strong while another organ might be too weak. For example, one person may be strong in the digestive function, but weak in the reproductive function. If your stomach is too strong due to overeating and you gain 30 or 50 pounds, this might weaken your sexual function or cause impotence. Eating a variety of foods can balance all the organs and help avoid overly nourishing any one organ.

Restore the body's balance in urgent conditions: When an individual is ill, the body's balance is temporarily lost. Readjusting the diet is required even though the body type is different. This means you need to be a little more flexible with body changes. For instance, if you are a Yang-type body constitution but caught a cold, your body temporarily changed to a Yin-type and you would feel better after having some ginger soup. If you are a cold-type body constitution but have a hemorrhoid relapse, you should still eat food with cold energy because you will become worse if you eat hot peppers, for example. In Western medicine, for example, sometimes in order to a save patient's life, the doctor has to open the patient's trachea even though it is invasive and dangerous. Please keep in mind: Always take care of whatever is urgent and important first, and then readjust whatever is needed later.

Eating the Right Foods

Eating the right food can sometimes help relieve different ailments. If you eat the wrong foods, the healing process slows down. The Chinese pay extreme attention to be sure they are eating the right foods to avoid overspending on medical bills. If you have dinner or lunch with Chinese people, you often hear them say "This is good for you, you should eat it." I think it is wise to eat the foods that are good for your health; but it is not just about medical expenses, it is about the quality of health and life.

Many Chinese use healing foods at the beginning of an illness, and use herbs when the illness becomes a little more advanced; they then use medication if the illness is severe. For instance, when the person is ill, Chinese eat rice porridge because the rice porridge is easy to digest and takes less energy to digest. It provides more energy available for healing.

Food is mostly used for relieving a mild ailment or in the beginning stages of an illness. If the illness goes too far and the condition becomes severe, food healing will not work; you need medical attention.

Common Colds ("Catch Cold")

- Avoid spicy and heavy foods (cheese, high portions of meat).
- Eat more liquid foods: thin oatmeal, porridge, chicken, or vegetable soup.
- Eat ginger scallion soup: 25g scallion heads (white and pale green parts), 25g fresh ginger, cook in two cups water for 5 minutes, and eat it before bedtime.
- Eat more fruits and vegetables.
- If there is also a headache, boil 10g peppermint and 10g crushed green onion heads with 1 cup water.
- If accompanied by a fever, eat foods with cold energy: mint tea, dandelion tea.
- If the cold is accompanied by a cough, cook orange peel in water and drink the brew. Alternatively, steam a pear with rocky candy inside the pear (cut pear in half and discard the core).

Diabetes

- Avoid refined sugar, fat, and overeating.
- Eat fresh corn, 100g every day.
- Make a sugar-free cake: 60 percent wheat bran, 40 percent wheat powder, egg.
- Eat all kinds of vegetables.
- Drink ginseng tea.
- Drink dandelion tea.
- Drink yarrow tea.
- Eat the pancreas of lamb, beef, or pork.

Hypertension

- Take seaweed and other sea vegetables.
- Boil peanuts, eat 30g or 40g a day, and drink the soup. Boil the peanut plant to make soup.
- Soak peanuts in vinegar for a week, eat 10 a day.
- Eat other foods: apple, celery, hawthorn berry, persimmon, watermelon, or use watermelon skin to make tea.
- Eat more food that can soften the blood vessels: kelp, sea grass, mung bean sprouts, fruits, less animal fat, and avoid egg yolk.

> As for myself, I dislike being sick, I do not like to go to the hospital, and I do not like to take pills. If I do not feel well, I will try anything natural to improve my condition. In 1995, when I was training and working in China to continue my education in TCM, I caught a cold, but I still had to work 12 hours a day. My brother-in-law cooked a nice ginger soup with scallions and black beans for me, and I felt better after eating it. Psychologically, I felt warm, cared for, nurtured, and loved.

Bronchitis

- Avoid cigarette smoking and alcohol.
- Drink honey lemon tea every day.
- Take 500g radish or daikon, 2 teaspoon honey, soak for 2 hours, then eat.
- Eat two walnuts per day.
- Slowly boil licorice root and orange peel for 15 to 20 minutes, and then drink the brew.
- Cut pear in half, put one tablespoon of "ice sugar" (white rocky candy), steam the pear, and then eat it and drink the juice.

Asthma

- Avoid dairy products; eat less sweets, meat, and fat.
- Eat smaller portions.
- Avoid smoking.
- Eat more carbohydrates from whole grain, food with a high content of fiber, vitamins, and minerals.
- Drink ginseng tea.
- Eat two walnuts every day.
- Eat daikon (radish family), 2-3 times a week.
- Drink honey lemon tea everyday.
- Eat fresh apricots.
- Drink licorice tea.

Anemia Due to Iron Deficiencies

- Eat spinach 2 or 3 times a week.
- Eat peanuts (with red coating) boiled with angelica roots.
- Boil 50g mung beans with 50g dried red dates, some brown sugar. Drink once a day.
- Eat the liver of beef, pork, lamb, or chicken.
- Eat whole grain foods.
- Take 300 mg vitamin C every day.
- Eat seaweed or sea vegetables.
- Eat more green leafy vegetables and sprouts.

- Eat Chinese red dates boiled with angelica roots.
- Eat royal jelly (bee pollen extract).
- Eat yams.

Skin Disease/Disorders

- Avoid alcohol, spicy food, fried food, and sweets.
- Avoid fish.
- Eat more leafy vegetables.
- Eat more carrots and celery without dip.
- Eat dandelions, as soup, salad, or stir-fry.
- Drink yarrow tea.
- Drink chrysanthemum tea every day.
- Eat mung bean soup.
- Drink green tea.
- Take Chinese herbal medicine (under the supervision of a TCM practitioner).

Goiter

- Bake 500g seaweed and 500g sea grass until dry, grind into powder, take 10g in warm water per day.
- Boil 10g seaweed and 10g kelp in water, make soup.
- Eat seaweed every day.

Ulcer or Gastritis

- Avoid spicy food, alcohol, coffee, deep fried food, acid food.
- Avoid overeating; eat small portions and soft food when you feel hungry; try not to eat when your stomach is still full.
- Eat a wide variety of cooked vegetables, avoid eating raw vegetables.
- Eat noodle soup with black pepper, in either meat or vegetable broth.
- Drink mild green tea every day.
- Eat more bean products, less meat.

Chapter 3

Healthy Balanced Diet and Weight Reduction, the Chinese Way

Chinese Healthy and Balanced Diet

In Chinese healing, we prefer a healthy and balanced diet rather than a macrobiotic diet. A Chinese healthy diet is slightly different from the macrobiotic diet. The macrobiotic diet excludes meat, whereas the Chinese healthy diet allows for small portions of a variety of meats. The Chinese healthy diet focuses on a balanced diet. The diet is based on eating whole foods, foods from natural sources (not chemically preserved), a variety of foods, ideal food portions (in moderation), and food in balance with one's body constitution. Eating food in harmony with nature and body constitution can help you avoid many health problems.

Eat whole foods: Eat foods as close to their natural form as possible. Eating primarily plant-based foods (low fat, no chemical additives) is always better. Unprocessed food is better than processed foods. This might be common sense to many people but, unfortunately, many people do not follow common sense, including me sometimes. We get accustomed to processed foods, fast foods, and refined foods; although these kinds of foods make our life easier, they have less nutritional value. We understand that the chemicals in the food could interfere with our body's normal chemical functions, but we often ignore this for the sake of convenience. The additives used in foods to preserve them can cause health problems if consumed in large quantities.

In my early years when I was in elementary school, I often ate whole foods due to the lack of food processing techniques in China; I hated to eat whole foods at that time. When the economy improved, people started to eat more processed and refined foods. From Yin-Yang philosophy, everything has two sides: the good side and the poor side. Whole foods might not taste as good, but they are much healthier than refined foods.

For example, unrefined flour has much more vitamin B_1, which has great value in maintaining good health. Vitamin B_1 promotes blood formation, carbohydrate metabolism, and production of hydrochloric acid, which is important in preserving good digestive function; which in turn has an impact on daily energy and immune function. Vitamin B_1 also optimizes cognitive activity and brain function. Moreover, Vitamin B_1 acts as an antioxidant that prevents body degeneration and aging.

Eat locally grown foods: Eating locally grown foods is better than eating foods from the other side of the state or country. Our body adapts to its local environment; our body more easily digests locally grown food. When we buy food from a local farm or pick it from our own garden, it tastes much better than what we get from the supermarket. The freshness of local foods means it has better nutritional value, too. We eat more local food in the summertime than in the wintertime; consequently, the energy level, in most people, is better during the summertime also.

Low calorie diet: In modern society, low calorie consumption is important for the adult diet in modern society. Nowadays, we eat too many calories, which we do not need to function. Most occupations require fewer calories, whereas most of us take in large amounts of calories that cause "traffic jams" in the body and contribute to many health issues.

Eat a variety: Eating a variety of foods can help us to maintain balanced health. From my years of clinical observations, picky eaters have much more imbalance than non-picky eaters (people who eat everything) do. These imbalances include either mental or physical problems. Common sense would tell us that eating everything will provide complete nutrition to the body; whereas, eating only certain foods would not provide complete nutrition and would cause an imbalance in the body. I have not conducted formal research on this subject, but my observations tells me that I would say the rate of mental illness (depression, anxiety, panic attack, ADD, OCD, etc.) is higher in people who are picky about the foods they consume.

Ideal food portions (eating in moderation): Eating food in moderation goes along with Chinese medicine's idea of "balanced health." As our economy improved, it did not reduce the number of patients making doctors' visits.

> Each year 62 million Americans are diagnosed with a digestive disorder. The incidence and prevalence of most digestive diseases increase with age. Notable exceptions are intestinal infections such as gastroenteritis and appendicitis, which peak among infants and children. Other exceptions include hemorrhoids, inflammatory bowel disease, and chronic liver disease, which occur more commonly among young and middle-aged adults.
>
> Women are more likely than men to report a digestive condition, particularly non-ulcer dyspepsia and irritable bowel syndrome (IBS). Whether women truly experience more troubles with their digestive systems than men is difficult to determine, but since women visit doctors more often

than they visit men, they have a greater opportunity to alert their doctors to their digestive problems. ... Gastroesophageal reflux disease (GERD) is a digestive condition that affects nearly one-third of the American population ... Inflammatory bowel disease (IBD) refers to two chronic intestinal disorders: Crohn's disease and ulcerative colitis. IBD affects between 2 to 6 percent of Americans or an estimated 300,000 to 500,000 people ... Irritable bowel syndrome (IBS) is a common functional disorder of the intestines estimated to affect 5 million Americans....

Peptic ulcer disease, estimated to affect 4.5 million people in the United States, is a chronic inflammation of the stomach and duodenum. Peptic ulcer disease is responsible for substantial human suffering and a large economic burden. Every year 4 million people report missing approximately 6 days from work because of their ulcers....

Digestive diseases cost nearly $107 billion in direct health care expenditures in 1992. Digestive diseases result in nearly 200 million sick days, 50 million visits to physicians, 16.9 million days lost from school, 10 million hospitalizations, and nearly 200,000 deaths per year.

The most costly digestive diseases are gastrointestinal disorders such as diarrheal infections ($4.7 billion); gallbladder disease ($4.5 billion); colorectal cancer ($4.5 billion); liver disease ($3.2 billion); and peptic ulcer disease ($2.5 billion).

Cancers of the digestive tract, which includes the colon, the gallbladder, and the stomach, are responsible for 117,000 deaths yearly. Noncancerous digestive diseases cause 74,000 deaths a year, with 36 percent caused by chronic liver disease and cirrhosis.

Of the 440 million acute noncancerous medical conditions reported in the United States annually, more than 22 million are for acute digestive conditions, with 11 million from gastroenteritis and 6 million from indigestion, nausea, and vomiting.

Digestive diseases have an enormous impact on health and the health care system in the United States. New technologies and new drugs have revolutionized the understanding and treatment of peptic ulcer disease and GERD. Successful outcomes of future research will hopefully continue to reduce the economic and health care costs related to diagnosing and treating digestive diseases.

(Above information was taken from National Digestive Diseases Information Clearinghouse)

Among the population at large, people eat too much food: 30 percent more food than necessary and 50 percent more in some people. The consequences are lethargy; weight, heart, high cholesterols, and elevated blood pressure problems; elevated blood sugar, fatty liver, PMS, fibromyalgia, lung problems, and so on. Some people succumb to stress eating, in which they use food to comfort and calm them. It is certainly the wrong way to deal with stress, because stress becomes even higher once other health issues develop. I hope this book can help these people avoid stress eating.

Food Balance and Body Constitution

As discussed above, for healthy people, using food to balance the body is not required, as long as they eat healthily. For people who have extreme Yin or Yang conditions that cause symptoms, using food to balance the condition is required. As also noted earlier, eat more Yin foods if you have too much Yang energy; eat more Yang foods if you have too much Yin energy.

If you are eating well all the time, then occasionally eating the wrong food will not harm your body. Our body recovers easily from temporary loss of harmony. If we eat the wrong foods all the time, then eating healthily occasionally will not help you to recover from the imbalance. The damage is already done; the imbalance will turn into a chronic condition, causing serious health problems. For instance, some people get sick around the holiday season from eating too much food, or the wrong foods. When they change back to their regular diet after the holidays, their body recovers. On the other hand, people who eat the wrong foods most of the time will always find it necessary to see doctors.

During the Chinese Cultural Revolution, I was sent to the countryside (farmland) because the Chinese government, at that time, sent all graduates to the countryside to experience farm labor, to learn how to be self-sufficient, and to appreciate hard work. I did a lot of hard physical labor planting trees, rice, corn, wheat, and other produce. We lived in very poor conditions, and we ate mostly vegetarian meals. We had meat once a week, which was a treat for us. Every few months, we went home where our parents often made meat dishes, and then put the food in jars for us to take to the farm. We ate only a little at a time, so that a jar of meat would last. We had no snacks, but we did drink tea every day. Our rice was from that year's harvest and it was the most delicious rice in the world. Our vegetables were from our own garden. For four years, we worked in the countryside, dealing with mud and bugs, poor hygiene, and hard physical labor, but we rarely got sick. I was healthy, despite the poor living conditions. My good health was most likely due to the fresh food, fresh air, healthy diet, and hard physical work. Was there stress? Yes! I was depressed because I could not use my talents, except for physical labor. I felt I was wasting my life in the country. I did not mind the physical work, but felt I could offer more than just labor. In the countryside or farmland, all foods were fresh and the water came from underground wells. I now appreciate the time I spent in the countryside, even though I hated it at the time. I learned so much, built stamina, experienced the beautiful places, people with beautiful hearts, and the best, healthy food. I learned how to farm, how to grow and harvest rice and wheat, how to deal with hard work, how to keep warm at night when there was no heat. I believe the old Chinese saying: "Without the bitter, you would not know the sweet." From hard times, I learned appreciation.

Recommended Healthy Chinese Diet

These are the recommended dietary proportions for people who would like to stay healthy and maintain optimum weight. This kind of low-calorie diet provides a better daily energy level, too.

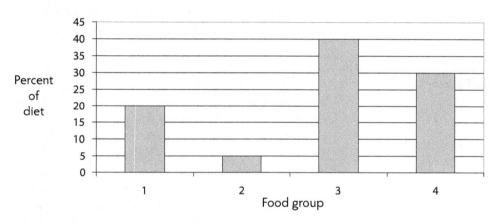

Group 1 is protein from various sources, such as meat, soy, etc.; should be about 20 percent.

Group 2 is miscellaneous foods, including healthy snacks, condiments; fats should be less than 5 percent

Group 3 is vegetables and fruits. It should be about 40 percent and includes all kinds of vegetables.

Group 4 is carbohydrates from grain or wheat products. It should be about 30 percent. These food categories are easily digested and absorbed.

You can use this kind of diet for three months. It might not be for everyone, but it is certainly good for many people.

Nutritional Value of the Healthy Chinese Diet

The Chinese healthy diet includes practically all kinds of foods, including whole grain and grain products, all wheat products, all kinds of vegetables and fruits, beans and sea vegetables, nuts and seeds, and fermented foods. It also includes meat products that provide high protein, amino acid, vitamins, and minerals. These foods are high in complex carbohydrates, fiber, vitamins, minerals, and other healthy elements.

Carbohydrates

Carbohydrates are a very important energy source. They are the most important source of energy in the diet of most organisms and are responsible for mediating intercellular communications.

Carbohydrates are easy to digest; they take less energy to digest than other parts of the diet. They slowly release calories, providing the body with long-lasting energy.

In China, a study of 400 Chinese centenarians revealed that every one of them ate rice and flour. In World War II, the Chinese Army fought against the Japanese for eight years with much hard work; they ate rice for every meal (sometimes only rice). There is much evidence that proves that complex carbohydrates give us long lasting energy.

People often ask me about the nutritional value in different kinds of rice. Some people believe that white rice is not good for health and causes weight problems; some even believe that white rice is toxic. I grew up eating white rice; sometimes three meals a day included white rice. I never knew about the brown rice until I came to United States in 1989 when I was 33 years old and weighed 110 pounds. Chinese people eat white rice at least once a day, but not many of them are overweight. If your vital energy and your diet are balanced, the food will not cause any problem. Only if your energy and diet are not balanced, then certain foods will cause problems. White rice is easier to digest than brown rice and it tastes good, too. If you have digestive problems, you should choose white rice, but white rice stimulates insulin release more quickly than brown rice. As we know, everything has two sides: the positive and the negative. Therefore, if you have a sensitive pancreas, you might choose a different kind of rice to eat, by comparing the different kinds of rice. Brown rice, millet, and whole grains release sugar more slowly than white rice, and the body does not release insulin as quickly. They provide energy slowly, which lasts longer, but white rice tastes much better and still provides plenty of energy for daily use.

In 2001, I took 16 people to China to see the beautiful parts of the country. We were hiking in the beautiful mountain in the area of Zhang Jia Jie in Hunan. We had to follow the path that was approximately 10,000 steps to the top of the mountain. We saw local men carrying people from bottom of the mountain to the top. A few of the people they carried were around 300 pounds. These men eat rice every day, and they looked very skinny. All of us wondered from where their energy and strength came.

Refined sugar releases energy in the body quickly, but it does not last long. It stimulates the pancreas to produce insulin quickly, causing low sugar response in the body, called hypoglycemia. The symptoms of hypoglycemia are sweating, weakness, hunger, dizziness, headache, and tachycardia, which could cause an overeating problem. The refined sugar burns quickly, which causes the body to store fat, and leads to weight gain.

Proteins

Protein is the best source of raw material for the vital processes of growth and repair in the body. It helps to build and renew cells, muscles, and tissues. Proteins are the building blocks of the human body. They are found abundantly in the muscles, tendons, blood, and organs. Hair, fingernails, and skin are all made of proteins. The antibodies of the immune system, most hormones, the hemoglobin of red blood cells, and all enzymes have protein as their basic component.

It is not just protein itself that we need in our diet, but the components known as amino acids. Of the 24 amino acids needed to maintain health, the eight known as the essential amino acids, can be obtained only from food. The body is able to manufacture the other proteins from amino acids and various substances.

The Chinese healthy diet supplies plenty of proteins, as well as the eight essential amino acids—more than enough to maintain body function. Whole grains, beans, sea vegetables, seeds, nuts, vegetables, fruits, and a little meat provide much of the protein the body needs. With a balanced diet that provides all kinds of amino acids, our body synthesizes the proteins to supply energy for bodily functions and daily activities. The protein synthesis and resynthesis are from amino acids of 125g to 220g of body protein each day. The protein requirement is higher in children due to their rapid growth. For example, adults require 0.8g of protein per kilogram of body weight, whereas infants need more than 2.0g per kilogram of body weight per day. It can be a little higher for people who have illness, such as metabolic dysfunction or injuries that require more protein for tissue repair.

Compare vegetable protein and meat protein; vegetable protein requires less energy to digest, whereas meat protein requires more energy to digest. The saturated fat in meat can be a potential cause of heart disease and other vascular problems. This is why I recommend eating meat in small amounts as a healthy way and better for the internal organs. Small portions of meat are more beneficial than no meat at all.

> "Eating a lot of protein, especially animal protein, is also linked to chronic disease. Americans consume a third more protein than the Chinese do, and 70 percent of American protein comes from animals, while only 7 percent of Chinese protein does. Those Chinese, who eat the most protein, and especially the most animal protein, also have the highest rates of the 'diseases of affluence' like heart disease, cancer and diabetes."
>
> (*New York Times* SCIENCE, May 8, 1990)

In the last 20 years, as the Chinese diet has changed to include more (meat) protein, health conditions have changed, too. Many more people suffer from heart disease now.

More cases of heart disease, hypertension, high cholesterol, cancer, and diabetes are now found in hospital visits. Many Chinese immigrants to the United States develop weight problems and high cholesterol due to changes in their diet. The health status of many American-born Chinese is not much different from Americans, because they eat the same food as other Americans.

Eating more vegetarian foods and less meat does not reduce the daily energy level and actually makes the energy last longer. Let us think about animals. Vegetarian animals like giraffes and antelopes have greater endurance than animals in the cat family. Tigers, who are meat eaters, take long, lazy naps after meals, because their energy has to be used for digesting the meat they eat.

Fiber

Standard American diets are extremely low in fiber. Many people think the fiber does not have nutritional value. Some food companies remove fiber from food, and then say it is high in nutrition. Once people see the foods they eat are supposedly high in nutrition, they assume they are eating healthily.

Actually, fiber affects the function of the entire digestive system, and is especially beneficial for the colon. It adds bulk to the feces, facilitating transit through the intestine. It dilutes the concentration of toxins, helping to prevent absorption of toxicity from depredated food, and protects the colon wall. High-fiber diets prevent bowel disease, colon cancer, constipation, hemorrhoids, diverticulitis, tooth decay (Oriental people have much less tooth decay, but more gum disease), diabetes, heart disease, blood pressure problems, cholesterol problems, and liver and gallbladder diseases. Many people take laxatives on a regular basis for symptomatic relief, but do not correct the problem. For people who have bowel problems, a change in diet is much better than taking a laxative that only helps to relieve the symptom temporarily; whereas, eating the right foods helps maintain normal bowel functionality in everyday life.

People who live in rural areas and regularly eat plenty of vegetables rarely have colon diseases. Colon disease is quite high in United States, especially colon cancer. According to data from American Cancer Society, the colorectal cancer is the third most common cancer diagnosed in men and in women in the United States. The American Cancer Society estimates that about 112,340 new cases of colon cancer (55,290 men and 57,050 women) and 41,420 new cases of rectal cancer (23,840 men and 17,580 women) would be diagnosed in 2007.

Colon disease and death from colon cancer can be significantly prevented if we eat the right diet. We need to educate our children about healthy diets that play an important role in preventing illnesses in adulthood.

Food containing fiber: There is an abundance of fiber on the outside surface of whole grains, seeds, beans, vegetables and fruits. For example, when we eat whole fruits, we will not lack fiber in our diet.[*]

---

[*] A comprehensive chart of food's fiber content from http://www.slrhc.org/healthinfo/dietaryfiber/fibercontentchart. html#fiber#fiber can be found online.

Fermented food: Americans eat much less fermented food than Asians. Fermented food is as important as fiber in keeping the intestines healthy. It produces lactic acid in the colon to maintain good bacteria and inhibit bad bacteria. Fermented foods include miso, pickles, fermented tofu and soybeans, soy sauce, yogurt, and so on. Westerners do eat a lot of yogurt, but the disadvantage of yogurt is that if the person has spleen energy imbalance, yogurt will not help the healing process; yogurt is too damp (i.e., causes water metabolism problems) and may cause weight gain and low energy.

Vitamins

Vitamins are organic compounds required by the body in trace amounts to perform specific cellular functions. They must be supplied to the body in the diet. Nine vitamins—thiamin, riboflavin, pyridoxine, cyanocobalamin, niacin, pantothenic acid, biotin, folic acid, and vitamin C—are water-soluble. Many of these provide cofactors for the enzymes of intermediary metabolism. These vitamins are not toxic; when ingested in excess of the body's needs, they are excreted in the urine. Four vitamins (A, D, E, and K) that are fat-soluble are stored in the liver and adipose tissue. An overdose of these vitamins can be toxic. These fat-soluble vitamins are digested, absorbed, and transported with the fat in the diet and are not excreted in the urine.

Vitamins contained in foods are listed in the table.

Table Vitamin Content and Their Functions in a Chinese Healthy Diet

Thiamine (Vitamin B_1)	Found in pork, whole grains, legumes, the outer layer of seeds, and whole wheat bread. Deficiencies of vitamin B_1 can cause skin problems, and somatic nervous system and central nervous system disorders.
Riboflavin (Vitamin B_2)	Found in milk, eggs, liver, and green leafy vegetables. The ultraviolet rays from sunlight can destroy riboflavin. Deficiencies of vitamin B_2 can cause cold sores on the lips and tongue, and dermatitis.
Niacin	Niacin is found in unrefined grains, cereal, milk, and lean meats, especially liver. A small amount of niacin can also be obtained from the metabolism of tryptophan. Niacin deficiencies can cause skin problems, gastrointestinal problems, and central nervous system disorders.
Pyridoxine (Vitamin B_6)	Good sources of vitamin B_6 are wheat, corn, egg yolks, liver, and meats. Deficiency of vitamin B_6 is rare but can be observed in infants fed with formula, women who take contraceptives, and alcoholics. The symptoms can be alopecia (hair loss) and other skin problems.
Biotin	Biotin is present in almost all foods, particularly liver, milk, and egg yolks. Most American diets are adequate in biotin; and since intestinal bacteria supply a large percentage of the biotin in the body, there is only a rare chance of biotin deficiency.

Folic Acid	It is found in green leafy vegetables, liver, lima beans, and whole grain cereal. Folic acid deficiency is probably the most common vitamin deficiency in the United States, particularly among pregnant women and alcoholics.
Cobalamin (Vitamin B$_{12}$)	Vitamin B$_{12}$ is present in liver, whole milk, eggs, oysters, shrimp, pork, and chicken. It can also be synthesized by natural bacteria in the digestive organs. A deficiency of B$_{12}$ from food is rare, but can be seen in people who have gastrointestinal problems, or have had part of their stomach and intestine removed. It can cause anemia and degeneration of nerve fibers.
Ascorbic Acid (Vitamin C)	Citrus fruits are rich in Vitamin C, as are potatoes (particularly their skins), tomatoes, and green leafy vegetables. Vitamin C deficiency can cause sore gums, loose teeth, fragile blood vessels, swollen joints, and anemia.
Carotene Vitamin A	Vitamin A is found in yellow and orange colored vegetables, leafy vegetables and fruits, liver, kidney, cream, butter, and egg yolks are also good sources of vitamin A. A deficiency of vitamin A can cause night blindness and dryness of the eye.
Vitamin D	Vitamin D can be found in fatty fish, eggs, liver, egg yolk, butter, and milk (in which vitamin D has been added). A vitamin D deficiency can cause demineralization of bone resulting in soft and pliable bones in children. In adults, it causes osteoporosis, which causes the bones to fracture easily. Vitamin D is the most toxic of all vitamins; therefore, an overdose should be avoided. Appropriate sunlight can be a good source of vitamin D, especially in the winter.
Vitamin K	Vitamin K is found in cabbage, cauliflower, spinach, egg yolk, and liver. There is also extensive synthesis of vitamin K by the bacteria in the intestines. A deficiency of vitamin K in adults is unlikely due to the synthesis of vitamin K by intestinal bacteria.
Vitamin E	Vegetable oils are rich in vitamin E and liver and eggs contain a moderate amount. A deficiency of vitamin E in the diet is rare. It is seen in adults with abnormal lipid absorption and transportation.

In the Chinese healthy diet, because the diet includes a variety of foods from all categories, it is not possible to have vitamin deficiency unless it is caused by a specific disease. If this is the case, you need help from a medical professional, either a Western or an Eastern practitioner.

Minerals

Minerals are inorganic elements that serve a variety of functions. They are cofactors in enzyme-catalyzed reactions, in the regulation of acid-based balance to keep normal blood pH, in nerve conduction and muscle irritability, and as structural elements in the body. They help maintain energy level, tranquilize the nerves, and maintain a healthy heart, healthy muscles, hair, blood, bone, teeth, and nails. With the Chinese healthy diet, it is rare to see mineral deficiency, due to the variety of food categories that contain a variety of minerals, vitamins, and amino acids. Taking mineral supplements without knowing what the body needs not only causes the body to absorb fewer minerals from food, but may also cause an imbalance of other minerals. Furthermore, an overdose of different minerals could cause other illnesses. For example, an overdose of calcium could cause kidney stones, an overdose of iron could cause hepatic carcinoma, and an overdose of sodium could cause hypertension and edema.

Among the mineral sources from food, sea vegetables contain the highest amounts of minerals. In an Asian diet, there is a much higher intake of sea vegetables than the typical American diet. As a result, mineral imbalance is rare in the majority of Chinese people.

Supplements

Vitamins and minerals have immense health benefits and help to maintain normal daily functioning. The Chinese healthy diet is high in vitamins and minerals. Sea vegetables, such as kelp and seaweed, are especially high in minerals. All fruits, vegetables and nuts, and seeds contain good quantities of vitamins and minerals.

A patient of mine, who worked in the health care field, came to see me eight years ago. Her complaint was about her stomach problem and low energy. She told me that she was bloated, had indigestion all the time, and sometimes diarrhea. She also told me that she took 10 different vitamins and minerals every day, and she was frustrated that she was still not feeling well. After I evaluated her with Chinese medicine techniques including looking at her tongue, checking her pulse, and palpating her stomach, I found out that her spleen and stomach energy were not working together, and her stomach energy was blocked. In terms of Western medicine, she had a mild inflammation in her entire digestive system. I told her that the first thing to do was to take fewer pills. I asked her to take one tablet each of a multivitamin and calcium per day, eat small portions during meals, and drink warm water. After several treatments and Chinese herbs, she recovered completely.

Another patient suffering from low energy and chronic sinus infection came to see me six years ago. He had to use antibiotics quite often, up to five times a year. He was only 35 years old, which I consider the most energetic stage of life. He told me he tried to exercise, such as working out in a gym, but had no energy to do it. He showed me the pills he took every day. The pills included all kinds of vitamins, minerals, antibiotics, supplements, and other health remedies. I counted 25 different pills. He was very anxious and asked me why he still felt lousy after taking such a variety of healthy supplements. After I evaluated him, I realized that his lung energy was weak to begin with, which could have been from a simple cold. He was also taking too many supplements that might have impaired his stomach energy; and the poor stomach energy could not support the lung; and the poor lung energy then affected the energy of the other organs, creating a vicious cycle.

I explained to him that if the Qi is not flowing well, no matter how much supplements he took, they would not help to heal. When he felt better after a few weeks' therapy, he could not believe it.

People who eat an assortment of these foods do not lack of vitamins and minerals. People who are picky eaters, who have digestion and absorption problems, who are on the road all the time, and do not allow time for eating good meals will have shortage in vitamins and minerals in the body, so they need vitamin supplements.

Many people assume that taking more supplements will make them feel better or heal them. True healing occurs when you take what you need, what your body lacks or needs. There is no evidence showing that extra vitamins give extra health benefits. You are just wasting money and energy. On the other hand, if you overuse vitamins and minerals, you might develop the symptoms related to vitamin overdose. Some people do need vitamins such as smokers and alcoholics, people using antibiotics or laxatives, and those who use certain medications that cause side effects in the digestive system.

If you are active, exercise regularly, eat well, eat a variety of foods, are physically in good shape, have good energy level, and a good mental spiritual status, sleep well, and are under 45, you do not need to take supplements. You are getting enough nutrients so your body functions well. Likewise, you do need supplements if you have some kind disorder or if you eat in extreme ways that causes an imbalance of nutrition and energy. The kind of supplements one should take depends on what kind problems you have. For example, if you do not eat enough fruits and vegetables, you need to take multivitamins daily; if you do not eat enough multigrain breads or cereals, or eat frozen food too often, you need vitamin B complex especially B_1. For mild problems, supplements might help, but only if you choose the right ones. If you have an organ energy blockage, the supplements will not work, because the supplements will not be digested and utilized. For mild energy blockages, simply adding appropriate exercise will help supplements work much better. For major blockages, you need treatment such as acupuncture or Chinese herbs prescribed by a practitioner.

Fats

The Chinese healthy diet does contain fats. Fat from plant sources contains more unsaturated fatty acids than those from animal sources. Most vegetable oils contain unsaturated fatty acids. Fatty acids can be oxidized by many tissues, such as liver and muscle, providing a source of energy. A small amount of animal fat is not harmful to the body; it is part of a normal dietary fat. We often think that cholesterol is bad for the body. Actually, cholesterol is the most abundant sterol in humans and performs a number of essential functions in the body. For example, cholesterol is a component of all cell membranes and functions as a precursor of bile acids, steroids, hormones, and vitamin D. Our body synthesizes cholesterol in the liver, intestine, adrenal cortex, and reproductive tissue including ovaries and testes. Only an excess of cholesterol or poor cholesterol metabolism can be harmful to our health, especially to our blood circulation system.

Dietary fat helps to absorb vitamins A, D, K, and E, which we need for maintaining normal metabolism in the body and preventing tissue degeneration.

Food Allergies

Living in the United States for 19 years, I have seen considerably more food allergy problems than in China. In general, the Chinese body type is more Yin and the American body type is more Yang. Yang-body types tend to have food allergies more often than the Yin-body types, especially when eating the wrong foods. From many years of clinical experience, I have observed that food allergies are most likely caused from consuming too much dairy, sugar, and meat. A hypersensitive body might also be inherited from parents who consumed too much dairy, sugar, and meat; these hypersensitive elements pass to their children though genes. Too much sugar intake from infancy and early childhood also increases food sensitivity. Too much dairy and sugar impairs spleen energy, which is related to digestion and absorption. Too much meat weakens stomach Qi due to overuse of this organ.

Dairy foods are high in protein and calcium, and are excellent food for human growth and tissue repair, but we do not need large amounts. Both dairy and sugar, if consumed to excess, cause dampness, which we call water retention, in the body. This leads to weight gain and digestive problems.

Meat contains high levels of proteins and amino acids, which are building blocks for proteins. Antigens and antibodies are made from protein. On the other hand, meat takes much more stomach energy to digest, so you have less energy for healing and daily activities. The more animal protein consumed in your diet, the higher incidence of hypersensitivity will occur in certain people. The hypersensitive part of the body can be located in the gastrointestinal tract, the skin, the respiratory system, etc. Too much meat is especially hard on the large intestine. The end substance from protein metabolism is nitrogen, which is toxic to the body. It causes bad smells when you pass gas; it also causes constipation, which makes you feel poorly if you do not move your bowels in several days.

Some people use the Atkins diet for weight reduction. It is a controversial diet. Since this diet involves high protein intake, it is believed to cause more harm to the body than good. During an experiment on high protein diets in mice, Chinese researchers used two groups of mice for the experiment. They put the first group of mice on a high carbohydrate and high fiber vegetarian diet; the second group ate a high protein diet. Three months later, they dissected the mice and found out that the vegetarian mice had normal brain tissue, but the high-protein mice showed brain atrophy under the microscope. These phenomena might occur in humans, too. In addition, protein digestion and degradation is handled by three different organs: the stomach, pancreas, and small intestine. A high protein diet could impair the function of these organs and cause various problems such as Crohn's disease, colitis, irritable bowel disease, gastritis, diabetes, low energy, and/or colon cancer. These diseases have a very high incidence in United States.

Maintaining Optimum Weight Naturally

Losing weight is not difficult, but maintaining optimum weight is a very difficult thing to do. For years, people have struggled with weight problems. In trying to lose weight, people go to dietary specialists, buy many dietary books trying to find answers, go to Weight Watchers, s try the Atkins diet, try vegetarianism, try to do more exercise, undergo surgery, and even starve themselves. Many of them lose weight from various practices, but they gain the weight back shortly after losing it. Some people developed other problems after trying special diets.

Weight problems have been an issue for years in the United States. From my years of experience in natural healing, I believe that two things are crucial: diet and lifestyle. Poor diet and a sedentary lifestyle are the primary cause of weight problems. There is another trigger factor that causes poor diet and immobile lifestyle, and that is stress. People who are stressed tend to eat poorly and exercise less, which leads to weight problems, and then consequently to many other problems.

Each individual has a different body type that makes some people lose weight more easily than others. One method that works well for one individual may not work for another person. After you have tried several ways to lose weight unsuccessfully, you might try the Chinese way; it is the healthiest way, and it works.

The most important thing in weight loss: What is most important for maintaining optimum weight in Chinese healing? It is your mind power.

Your mind produces intention; your intention creates your goal and determination, and then directs your positive behavior. As long as your mind is there, your positive behavior will guide you to the optimum weight.

Let us do a thought experiment: Imagine that you are going to have Swiss chocolate in about 2 minutes…. What do you feel? Your mind anticipates the pleasurable experience of eating the delicious chocolate. Now imagine that you are going to have ravioli made from worms and flies in about 2 minutes…. What do you feel? You might want to vomit. Do you see the difference? There is a huge mental change between these two images, which you rarely ever realize. If someone told you the food you are about to eat was poisonous, of course you would not eat it. We get information from what we see and what we hear, but the most important information that we should get is from what we experience. Without experience, our information is incomplete.

Having a healthy and determined mind for weight reduction is extremely important. This is the key to success. People who set a goal with a determined mind tend to be able to lose and maintain weight. People who make excuses tend to have less success losing weight. Humans have a hard time rejecting food, especially delicious food. From Yin-Yang philosophy, we learn that food can be our friend and our enemy, too. If your mind is healthy and positive, you know when to stop eating; if your mind is weak, you might use food to cover up some other issue or stress, and continue to eat until your stomach is overfull, which is what creates weight problems and health issues.

Try to think differently about food.

"It is tasty and I really want it, but if it is not healthy, I decide not to eat."

"I'd rather keep my health instead of pleasing my mouth."

"Lose weight for health, not just for looks."

"I'm not going to have dinner tonight because it is too late; it is not good for my health if I eat a big dinner this late."

"If I lose my health, it will cost me much more; it is not worth eating unhealthy food."

"Life is too short; I'd like to stay healthy and enjoy my life."

You have to decide what is important to you. Is your enjoyment of food most important or is your weight and health more important? If you do not care about your health, and just want to enjoy each moment of eating, that is fine, it is your choice. You might choose this as part of your way of enjoying life, but some people choose to be healthy. In China, it is tradition to choose foods with good nutrition, to do exercises to keep the body fit, and to take herbal tonics to live longer. I cannot say all of these are right, but the most important thing is to have a mind focused on good health.

What do you really want?

If you are certain that health and weight are more important to you than food, you then set up a goal and work toward it. If you do not reach your goal by the time you set, set up another one. Each person's body is different, and some people are able to lose weight on time while others need more time and discipline. You should not be disappointed when you see other people lose weight sooner than you do. As long as you are faithful about your work and your choice, you will reach your goal. You can do it. Just do whatever is important to you.

Weight reduction requires discipline. The best way is to work in a group. I had several weight-reduction classes at my clinic. Even after just 10

I had a patient who came to me for help with her weight problem. It was the end of May, and she wanted to be thin during the summer so she could look nice and wear a bathing suit at the beach. After I told her about the importance of eating the right foods and the discipline associated with eating, I asked her, "what is more important to you during summer vacation — weight or food?" She told me that she would not give up her enjoyment of food because she did not want to have that discipline in her diet during summer vacation. I told her it might be difficult but when she is ready, she should start losing weight in the fall. The point of this story is that you have to know what is important to you in your life.

weeks, and only one class per week, everyone who was overweight and followed the instructions from the class lost between 5 and 15 pounds. Best of all, they felt better than before, and their energy level was much higher. Of course, if you have good discipline, you do not have to work with a group.

Golden Tips for Weight Reduction

In order to make it clear what is involved in losing weight, I have summarized some tips for health and weight reduction. Try them for 10 weeks; you might be surprised by the results.

Keep healthy diet habits, eat a variety of foods

In Chinese healing, eating only certain foods that overly nourish one organ might cause some other organ imbalance. Eating a variety of foods will help to build a well-balanced body. These should include foods you like and do not like. All foods have nutritional value. You eat for health, not just for pleasing your mouth. You might like it later. I used to hate turnips, but at one Thanksgiving dinner, I forced myself to eat some because I knew the turnip has great nutritional value. After awhile, I started liking it. In Yin-Yang philosophy, everything has two sides: food tasting good can cause overeating and weight gain; food that does not taste as good but is nutritious might help you to lose weight. Life always balances itself.

When you are hungry, try not to eat the foods you love, because you will definitely eat more than usual. You should try to eat food you do not like particularly (yet that has good nutritional value) when you are hungry. This is one way to prevent overeating. In addition, the food you do not like would taste better to you at this time.

Do not buy unhealthy food you crave

Most people like sweets, and if you have one chocolate, you will most likely want another one or two. However, if you do not have any, you will not think about it. In this way, you can start the habit of not buying these foods. Even though some publications state that chocolate is healthy for the body, it is not healthy if you eat too much of it. Having chocolate (e.g., ice cream) occasionally will not cause weight gain. Nevertheless, when you always buy it and eat it regularly, you most likely will gain weight.

Do not go food shopping when you are hungry

In the past, every time I went food shopping when I was hungry, I regretted it. First, I spent more money than usual. I also bought more food that tasted good but was not healthy. Finally, I overate, sampling various foods until I was stuffed. I then felt bloated and terrible. When you are so hungry, everything in the supermarket looks good to you. Your craving overpowers your wisdom; you lose your discipline and mind power. Therefore, the best time to go food shopping is when you are full, which is when you are more likely to buy what you need, not whatever you see.

Start healthy diets at a young age

Poor diet can cause obesity and other health problems later in life. Many families overly nourish children when they are young with too much food, too much fat and sweets, and not enough vegetables, fruits, and food from different categories. When my kids were young, they had friends who would come to our house for dinner and to sleepover. I was surprised that most of them did not eat vegetables and fruits. I would sometimes force them to eat them, but it did not really work, because they still ate the same way when they went home. Many kids, including mine, like pizza, hamburgers, French fries, cheese, and sweets. Eating these foods very often contributes to disease later in life such as allergies; high cholesterol; bowel disease; heart disease; hypertension; and gallbladder disease; low immune function; and other ailments. We need to educate our children about healthy diets, but the first step is to educate ourselves. Children learn many things from parents, even if they do not realize it at the time. You still remember many things they taught you.

Reduce meal size

A researcher in China did an experiment on mice on two groups of mice; one group ate as much as it wanted with no control on the quantity or the times at which the mice ate; the other group ate small portions only during specific times. After several months, the group that ate large quantities of food died sooner than the group on the controlled diet. The results showed that overeating shortened their lifespan.

We generally eat too much food, especially at dinnertime. This is related to our lifestyle; we do not have much time in the morning and at noon, so we have to enjoy our large and delicious meal at night, when we have time to cook, eat, and relax. There are two health hazards from eating large meals at night. The first one is the large portion causes impairment of stomach Qi, which leads to digestive problems; the second is that we do not have much activity to stimulate our circulation at night. Our metabolism is slower during the night than in the daytime. Any fat we ingest tends to be stored in the body and causes weight gain. The fat can also build up in vascular walls, which leads to heart disease, hypertension, arthrosclerosis, diabetes, and low energy. Just think about how we feel after Thanksgiving dinner: tired, sleepy, and bloated, so that we still feel fatigued the next day. It is just like overeating at a buffet at a restaurant after which we do not feel well for several days.

Chinese medicine explains that the large portion of food will take more energy from your body to digest; you are overloading the digestive system just as you might overwork your body. Appropriate work is good for the body, whereas overwork will damage the body. Your stomach is the same way. When you feel full, it is time to stop eating. If you continue to eat, you start to overload. Observations on many people who lived longer lives show that eating small portions leads to longevity and healthy bodies. This is especially true for ill people; eating small portions can conserve the body's energy for healing. If you are growing, your metabolism is high, and you do need more food; but for adults who do not grow any longer, the food we eat is for maintaining daily energy levels and body functions. Adults can get enough nutrition from a small, balanced meal. In this country, most occupations do not require much physical work; adults or older people do not burn as many calories as younger people. Active children need to eat more food because they burn more energy.

I have experimented on myself by eating large portions of food for a while to see how I feel; I then eat small portions of food to see how I feel. I eat certain foods to experience the results, and then stop eating these foods to experience different results. That was how I found out the truth in my own dieting. Because each individual is different, you might have a different experience. If you occasionally have a big meal (which we all do), skip your next meal or eat very lightly at your next meal. This way, you give your digestive system a little break to avoid energy blockage. You can do self-examination to find out if you have a blockage in your digestive system by putting pressure on the stomach after eating. Pain over the stomach area indicates that your digestive system is not very healthy.

If you do physical work that burns more calories, you can eat larger quantities of food; whereas, if you have a sedentary lifestyle, in which you do not burn so many calories, you need to reduce the size of the portions you eat.

Avoid eating late

You do not have to have a real meal if you come home late. The necessity of a real meal is all in your mind. If your mind tells you that you must have a real dinner everyday, you will eat a large dinner everyday. If your mind tells you that you can have very light food for dinner, you will then be able to control your weight. A light dinner might be a salad, or a vegetable, a piece of fruit, or crackers, nuts, or soup, and so on. If your mind says so, dinner can be anything, as long as it stops the hunger. Eating late can cause many physical problems. Normally after dinner, our activities are limited. Most people just relax and watch TV, talk, or read a book. Rarely do people go out to start physical work. Shortly after eating the big meal, it would be bedtime, when your metabolism is slower. Your blood circulation is also slow. Any food, plus dessert, plus snack, all these calories and fat would go through your body slowly. The cholesterol and fat tend to deposit on your arteries. After years of this, your artery walls get thicker and thicker. Eventually, an artery may become completely closed, and when this happens, you could have a heart attack or stroke. If you are lucky, the doctor can save your life.

If you come home late, you should skip dinner; just have a little something to eat, just to fill your stomach. The food should contain very few calories. I often come home late, but most times, I just have a small portion of something such as soup, vegetables, a few noodles, or a salad. I understand the consequences if I eat a "real" dinner. Only occasionally will I have a big meal with friends late at night.

Avoid being too hungry

If you feel hungry and wait too long to eat, most of the time you will not stop eating until you are completely stuffed. When you are too hungry, you do not eat slowly; when you slow down, it means you are overfull. Your brain does not get the "full" signal until you are overfilled, and then it is too late. A healthy snack between meals can prevent hunger and overeating. Furthermore, if you are too hungry before going to bed, low blood sugar could affect your sleep. However, both high blood sugar and low blood sugar can affect your sleep. Therefore, neither being overly hungry nor overly full is ideal.

I recommend that you always keep some nuts or trail mix with you. Eat several nuts or dry fruits one hour before your next meal, or you can eat fruits or vegetables instead. This way you will not be so hungry and overeat during regular meals.

Arrange three meals wisely

Breakfast: Breakfast should be a small portion of something healthy. In the morning, your digestive system is not completely awake yet, so you do not need to eat a large portion, unless the meal is late morning brunch. Since you need various nutrients, you should change the menu for breakfast each day. For instance, you might have oatmeal one morning, an apple or other fruits plus some nuts the next morning, whole grain toast on the third day, an egg on the fourth day, a bagel on the fifth day, cereal on the sixth day, and an omelet on the seventh day. This way, you include all of the nutrition the body needs.

Lunch: You should really enjoy your meal at lunchtime. You can eat pretty much anything, but adults should eat low-fat foods. Lunch is during the day, when you are active, so you have much more opportunity to burn calories. For this reason, lunch should be your most important and enjoyable meal. Unfortunately, many people do the opposite and eat a very light lunch.

Dinner: For most Americans, dinner is the most important/largest meal of the day. Nevertheless, this is the daily meal that requires the most attention in order to maintain good health and weight. At dinnertime, you should eat a well-balanced meal in moderate portions. Your dinner should be low in fat and low in sweets. After dinner, you should not have dessert except perhaps a piece of fruit. Eating cake, pastry, or other heavy sweets for dessert is unhealthy in many ways. Many people eat a large dinner and eat small portions during their other meals. Over time, you will most likely develop ailments.

Manage stress

Many people eat more and eat the wrong food when they are stressed. They use food to de-stress their life. According to Chinese medicine, stress can cause energy blockages in the organ system, such as the liver, spleen, heart, and kidneys. When one organ has a blockage, the blockage will soon affect another organ. Therefore, if a person's stress is prolonged, this person will soon have some kind of health issue. Chinese healing art and culture has many ways to help manage stress and restore the balance of the organs. First, you can learn Daoist techniques to relax your body and mind. Furthermore, you can undergo some acupuncture that unblocks energy so that your body relaxes itself, thus enabling you to avoid a negative cycle that worsens your health. Studying Daoist philosophy can be helpful in stress management because it helps you clear the clutter from your mind, understand Yin-Yang, nature, and a spontaneous lifestyle. Once your mind is clear, you know will know what to do. Your next step could be to start Taiji practice, along with daily meditation. Daily meditation could be just five minutes each day. There are many other ways to manage your stress and many resources are available from books and the Internet.

> A friend of mine is a Western health care practitioner, who works very hard in the hospital, eats no breakfast and no lunch, but has a very large dinner every night. He not only has a weight problem, but also has a heart condition for which he takes baby aspirin everyday, along with other pills, such as for cholesterol and blood pressure. He uses the medication to maintain his daily functions because he will not change the way he eats. Evidently, the amount of stress he has to deal with prevents him from changing his habits.

Burn more calories

Spicy food helps to burn calories. Power walking or other fast-paced exercise also helps to burn calories. Some people do not like to sweat; however, sweating from a workout is beneficial because it means that you actually have had an effective workout, your metabolism is fast, and you are losing water through your skin. I love hiking, and if I hike two days in a row, my weight drops between 3 and 5 pounds.

Avoid drinking soft drinks

Research shows that drinking soft drinks causes weight gain. Most soft drinks contain a significant amount of sugar. In general, we consume more sugar than we need even without soft drinks, such as sugar in coffee, pastry, meals, tea, bread, snacks, and at meals, etc., which is partly the cause of weight problems. No matter how well you eat, you will not lose weight if you drink soda on a regular basis.

Weight Control Program—Food and Exercise Log

Using these logs to boost your discipline can help you watch your progress. You can see the relationship between your discipline and weight. You can also trace previous health conditions so you see the difference in your health before and after going on this kind of diet. If you already have a strong mind focused on a healthy diet, you might not need these logs, but for beginners, it is a good way to start your journey.

Weight Control Program I

Table Pre-Program Form

Name	
Commonly used foods in the past (food I love or eat a lot)	
Cravings	
Disliked food (The foods I hate or avoid)	
Daily or regular exercise	
Health concerns	
Other regular activities	
Other foods or junk foods	
Daily drinking habits (soda, water, juice, etc.)	
My present weight	

This log can help you record the history of your health and lifestyle. Fill it out before you start the program. After three months, check the log again to see what has changed.

Weight Control Program II

Homework with Food and Exercise Log

Name: _____   Start Date: _____

Week 1:

	Monday	Tuesday	Wednesday	Thursday	Friday	Saturday	Sunday
Breakfast							
Lunch							
Dinner							
Snacks							
Exercise							

Weight/Notes:_____

Week 2:

	Monday	Tuesday	Wednesday	Thursday	Friday	Saturday	Sunday
Breakfast							
Lunch							
Dinner							
Snacks							
Exercise							

Weight/Notes: _____

Week 3:

	Monday	Tuesday	Wednesday	Thursday	Friday	Saturday	Sunday
Breakfast							
Lunch							
Dinner							
Snacks							
Exercise							

Weight/Notes: _____

Week 4:

	Monday	Tuesday	Wednesday	Thursday	Friday	Saturday	Sunday
Breakfast							
Lunch							
Dinner							
Snacks							
Exercise							

Weight/Notes: _____

Week 5:

	Monday	Tuesday	Wednesday	Thursday	Friday	Saturday	Sunday
Breakfast							
Lunch							
Dinner							
Snacks							
Exercise							

Weight/Notes: _____

After the fifth week, you might have developed the discipline, which you will automatically use to eat the right foods and drink the right liquids in the right amounts. If you are still having weight problems, you might consider TCM care such as acupuncture or certain herbs to balance your energy.

See Appendix 2 with a variety of helpful TCM recipes.

Chapter 4

Chinese Exercises for Healing, Disease Prevention, and Good Health

"There is a doctor inside each patient. Let us give the doctor who resides inside a chance to go to work"   —Albert Schweitzer, MD

For centuries, the ancient Chinese used natural body movements to fight disease. These movements are still very popular in China due to their effectiveness in human healing and disease prevention. Worldwide popularity has been increasing each year.

There is an old saying, "The time to repair the roof is when the sun is shining." When I was a young girl, my grandmother often told me "you should always dig the well before you are thirsty," which certainly indicates the importance of preventive work.

Early every morning, in China's parks and other public places, people practice a beautiful dance-like exercise to music provided by portable CD players. They practice various forms of Taiji, Qigong, and other exercises. Most do it to prevent disease, others do it for healing. Even though many have health insurance, they prefer to keep in good health. Moreover, they want to feel good, to stay full of energy, and able to do things they like to do. In addition, they like to do things to allow them to live longer: eating and drinking well, taking certain supplements, doing healthy activities, and having social commitments.

Self-healing is a big part of the Chinese lifestyle. Every year when I visit China, I go to the parks to watch the thousands of people who are exercising. It is so much fun to watch them. Even in bad weather, hot or cold, people still exercise outside their homes. Many Chinese believe the only way to stay healthy is to maintain good Qi, which is the source of everything.

Self-healing involves different components, not just one or two. In order to do self-healing, one must develop healthy habits and be able to change and adapt

117

About six years ago, I was experiencing many problems: headache, insomnia, back pain, bronchitis, hip pain, leg injury, anxiety, and asthma. Thinking I had meningitis, I went to an emergency room for my severe headache where I waited 45 minutes; no one paid any attention to me. I told the nurse I had an unbearable headache. All she said to me was, "The doctors are too busy now," I could not wait any longer so I went home, treated myself with acupuncture, and took aspirin. This experience certainly convinced me to do the best I can to avoid going to a hospital again.

In most cases, I prefer a natural way of healing unless I need to use an antibiotic to stop an infection. I would definitely take medication if I had a serious disease or life threatening illness; however, I do everything in a natural way and I use self-healing on a daily basis. From all these years of practice and experience, I can design different self-healing prescriptions for different problems, including diet, exercise, positive outlook/attitude, and so on. I do this for patients and for myself. I am now free of most of my problems. If I lose my discipline, I know I will digress and my problems will reappear. If I eat or drink too much, I know I will suffer the next day. Self-healing involves hard work, effort, and discipline; but I stick to it, because I hate to be sick, and I would hate to lose my energy and enjoyment of life. I love life. There is still so much I want to do and enjoy. Without good health, I would not be able to do so, which is why I hope you will enjoy the benefits of self-healing.

to something different. If you do not want to change, the practice of self-healing will be difficult. For instance, very tight muscles cause discomfort. In order to feel better, you need to do certain exercises to loosen your muscles. Acupuncture treatments can help you loosen your muscles, but without certain types of exercise, your muscles will tighten again after awhile. When one of my patients suffers from bowel problems, I ask them to change to a diet that harmonizes the digestive organ; however, if they do not want to change their diet or give up the food that is causing the problem, then the symptoms can become worse, and they will most likely heal poorly.

Chinese Exercises for Healing and Disease Prevention

The Chinese have been using exercise for healing and disease prevention for about 4,000 years. In an underground tomb from West Han dynasty (206 B.C.), a painted fabric chart showing groups of human figures in different fundamental exercise poses. The poses form basis for many different types of Qigong exercises, which are still widely practiced by a large numbers of Chinese. This finding proved that our ancestors began using exercise to maintain health at least 2,000 years ago. Worldwide, people are now seeing the benefits of Qigong and Taiji.

Chinese exercise originated during a time when many people were very sick and very poor. China has had epidemic outbreaks of disease in its history, but people learned from their experience with high mortality. They realized they could reduce the death rate if they kept their bodies moving because medicines were not very effective at that time.

Benefits of Chinese Exercise

Cardiovascular benefits: Qi is dynamic, a motor that pushes the blood to where it should go. If the Qi is strong and circulates well in the body, the blood also circulates well in the body. If the Qi is stagnated, or weak, the blood also stagnates. Chinese exercise balances the body's chemicals, which is important to maintain a healthy heart and blood pressure. There is much less heart disease in China. Not only does diet play an important role, but also the Chinese tradition of regular exercise contributes to better heart health. Chinese exercise enhances autonomic function, in particular activating the vagus nerve, which is an excellent way to preserve heart energy.

Respiratory benefits: Through deep and slow breathing, more oxygen goes into the lungs and blood. More oxygen goes to the brain, too. The increased oxygen helps to improve defensive energy, which in Western medicine is called the respiratory immune system. If your respiratory immune system is strong, it indicates that your immunoglobulin A (IgA) is normal, and you will have fewer chances of getting colds and other respiratory infections. IgA is an antibody in the respiratory tract, which protects

> My father had a severe lung disease. I also have had asthma, but I use an inhaler only occasionally when the weather changes, if there is poor air quality, or if I run in cold weather. There have been times when I have had to go to the ER in the middle of the night due to an asthma attack. However, most of the time, I do not have symptoms, which gives me even more incentive to practice Chinese exercise regularly.

the respiratory tract from various germs or pathogens; that is why students who practice Taiji or Qigong regularly tell me that they have not been sick for a long time.

Gastrointestinal (GI) benefits: Taiji and Qigong can improve stomach and spleen energy, which is related to digestion and absorption. Some Qigong includes self-massage around the stomach to help digestion. With regular practice, your GI enzymes and GI mobility will maintain their normal functions. Furthermore, regular practice helps you to maintain the optimum weight for your body.

Musculoskeletal benefits: From improved Qi and blood circulation, your muscles receive more oxygen, good muscle resiliency and muscle tone results, your joints become more flexible than a non-practitioner's, and muscle degeneration is delayed as you age. You maintain a younger body even though you are becoming older.

For muscle strength and muscle mass, weight lifting is still better, unless you do martial arts weapon exercises. Most practitioners use Qi (energy) rather than their muscles.

Central nervous system benefits: From improved Qi and balance of the body chemicals and neurochemicals, your concentration and mental alertness improve, and the mind remains sharp for a long time. You will most likely have less depression, anxiety, stress, and confusion, and you will be more focused. Chinese exercise helps to improve memory, quickens response to learning, and improves the ability to perform daily tasks with great ease. Because Chinese exercise is related to various kinds of learning, it is an excellent way to delay the brain's aging. It also helps to preserve vision and hearing during the aging process.

Metabolism and endocrine system benefits: Once your Qi is balanced, your metabolism most likely stays normal. Over time, even high cholesterol levels drops after practicing regularly. A type of Taiji (16-step Taiji for healing) does wonders for hormonal imbalance, giving you immediate relief.

Immune system benefits: Chinese exercise does an excellent job of maintaining good immune system function, as can be seen during flu seasons. During flu seasons, while many people become sick; those who practice Chinese exercise (especially Qigong) regularly remain healthy. If you stop practice, however, your immune system changes, too. Chinese exercise is excellent for assisting cancer healing due to improved immune function and strengthened organ energy from Qi practice.

Other benefits: Delay aging, improve balance, reduces risk of falling and injury.

As can be seen, there is much evidence that shows that Chinese exercises are excellent workouts for preventing illness and delaying aging. There are many different forms of Chinese exercise, such as Taiji, Qigong, martial arts, and various meditations. There are exercises that focus on an internal energy workout, while others focus on an external energy workout. From a healing point of view, the exercises that focus on internal energy are preferred. Furthermore, the people who are most in need of healing are older, and it is better for older people to do internal exercises. The external exercises, such as certain martial arts, are better for the younger population. That is why martial art practitioners often change their practice to Qigong or Taiji when they become older. Internal energy workouts include Taijiquan, Qigong, Baguazhang, Xingyiquan. In this book, however, we focus on Qigong and Taiji.

Chinese Exercises for Good Health

When compared with Western exercise, we find that many Chinese exercises work on internal energy, whereas many Western exercises work on external energy. You should choose whatever exercise you like and do it regularly. Some of the difference between Chinese exercise and Western exercise are indicated below.

Chinese Exercise

1. Improves energy circulation, flexibility.
2. Movements are slow, gentle; looks as if you are not exercising. Nevertheless, you feel very good afterwards, emotionally, mentally, and physically.
3. Correct breathing is important because it is related to internal energy.
4. There are no age limits, no restrictions.
5. Improves posture in certain exercises.
6. Fun to learn; sometimes challenging, which is good for preventing aging of the brain.
7. As you become older, you perform better in certain exercises (Taiji and Qigong, but not fast martial arts). Nevertheless, the exercise is good for all age groups, not limited to seniors.
8. Mind/body connection involved.
9. For both health maintenance and healing of illness; closely related to longevity.
10. It is more a Yin-type exercise.

Western Exercise

1. Workout improves muscle mass and muscle tone, does little on flexibility.
2. Improves circulation by increasing heart rate.
3. Movements are fast, heavy, vigorous.
4. More focus on external energy.
5. More focus on physical body, less on mind.
6. There is an age limit; fewer choices when you are older.
7. Some restrictions for people who have certain medical conditions.
8. For health maintenance, not for healing.
9. Suitable for the younger generation.
10. It is a more Yang-type exercise.

Being active is not enough to prevent illness; it is not the same as regular exercise, either. On the contrary, you lose more than you gain by being active without the balance of Yin-Yang. You might know some people who are very busy but have many physical problems. If you have "balanced busyness" in your life, the chances of being sick will decrease.

I have discussed both types of exercises, both of which are important in our lives. They complement and balance each other. One is not better than the other is; they are just different.

Table Differences between Chinese Exercise and Western Exercise

	Chinese Exercise (Qigong and Taiji)	Western Exercise (Weight lifting, aerobic, treadmill, etc.)
Purpose	For health maintenance, disease prevention, and healing of illnesses. Leads to longevity.	For health maintenance, disease prevention, not for healing. Not much relationship to longevity.
Cost effectiveness	Most inexpensive. Does not require special place and equipment.	Can be expensive. Some exercise regimes need special place and equipment.
Mind and body benefits	Lasts longer. Meditation manifested through the physical movement; very pleasurable.	Short-term effects. Most types of workouts are physical; can also be pleasurable.
Autonomic nervous system involvement	Stimulates parasympathetic nerve system, considered/act as a natural tranquilizer.	Stimulates sympathetic nervous system, considered/act as a natural stimulant.
Breathing	Requires special breath training.	Normal breathing based on exertion and type of exercise.
Body parts involved	Whole body, including enhancement of immune system.	Partial, depends on the type of exercise.
Oxygen consumption	Consumes less oxygen.	Consumes more oxygen.
Learning involved	Yes, very much so. Good for preventing aging of the brain.	Some yes, some no.
Circulation	Improves internal energy flow that promotes blood circulation. (Qi is the commander of the blood; blood is the mother of the Qi. A different approach working on circulation.)	Increases circulation by increasing heart rate from various physical workouts.
Muscles	More focus on working to improve flexibility, core strength, and muscle resilience.	Focus is on muscle mass, muscle tone, muscle strength, a little less on flexibility.
Movements	Movements are slow, gentle but powerful. Serious learning and practice is required. Structural, involves learning and coordination.	Aerobic movements, fast, heavy, vigorous, easy to learn, and easy to do. Repetitive. Some demand less from coordination.
Energy aging	Qi stays the same even with aging.	Strength decreases with aging.
Energy focus	Focus on internal energy.	Focus on external energy.
Limitations	Generally speaking, no limitations, no restrictions, except for fast martial arts. (The older you are, the better you are.)	There is age and condition limitations, some restrictions (e.g., bad knee, hypertension, cannot do fast running). (The older you are, the worse off you are.)

	Chinese Exercise (Qigong and Taiji)	Western Exercise (Weight lifting, aerobic, treadmill, etc.)
Group energy	Big part of the practice.	Only in some sports. Most of the time, groups are not involved.
Participants	With or without health problems, for all ages.	Mostly healthy people, but it can be for all.
Other	Positive addiction (people love it!), attractive, challenging, no special needs, social, entertainment value in certain forms, mind/body exercise.	Some sports are addictive and have entertainment value.

Qigong and Taiji Practice

Differences between Taiji and Qigong

Many people are aware of Taiji (Tai Chi), but not Qigong. Maybe there is more publicity about Taiji than Qigong. People have asked me about the difference between Taiji and Qigong. The relationship between Taiji and Qigong is that Qigong is a beginner-level internal energy workout and Taiji is an advanced, internal energy workout. To understand this, one must try them first and then practice both for a while.

Taiji and Qigong practice both work to improve the energy flow in the body, harmonize body and mind, reduce stress, and prolong life. Both can be used for assisting self-healing. There are, however, important differences:

Table Differences between Taiji (Tai Chi) and Qigong

Taiji	Qigong
Advanced energy workout.	Beginner energy workout.
Needs full concentration.	At times, Qigong requires a little less than full concentration.
Movements, which are slow and circular, may initially be difficult, and take a long time to learn well.	Movements are simple, easy to follow, easy to learn, and often are repetitive. Some Qigong involves self-massage.
Five main styles or forms with other variations.	Five categories, but more than a hundred forms.
Breathing is slow and deep, coordinated with each movement.	Breathing can be slow or fast. It varies in different forms; breath is also coordinated with each movement.
Is a martial art, but also a natural medicine.	Is a natural medicine, and used to enhance martial arts skills.
Most practice occurs in a walking motion.	Can be practiced in any position.
Not practical for severely ill people.	Good for all kinds of illness, no restrictions.

Taiji	Qigong
Beginners may become easily frustrated.	Some people may find it too simple.
See results only after a long while.	See results more quickly.
It Is a type of self-discipline.	It is self-therapy.
Practitioners are usually younger people, but is for everyone.	Practitioners can be older, but it is for everyone.

Qigong

For many centuries, Chinese people have used Qigong (Qi Gong) as an exercise to prevent illness and maintain good health. It has a long history of being used as a healing modality. Despite this history, Qigong still seems mysterious to many Americans.

The word Qigong is made up of two words, *Qi* (氣) and *Gong* (功). Qi is usually translated as energy, vital energy, or life force. It is the energy that underlies everything in the universe. The word Gong can be translated as skill practice or workout to reach the level. The word Qigong conveys the meaning of practice concerned with exercising the Qi or as an energy workout. The use of Qigong to improve and maintain health was first mentioned in the *Huang Di Nei Jing*, known in English as *The Yellow Emperor's Classic of Internal Medicine*, written about 200 B.C., thus proving that Chinese ancestors used Qigong for healing and disease prevention. Through this kind of internal energy workout, our body and mind becomes easily and quickly connected, and our body's organ systems begin to self-regulate and start working to balance our body chemicals in all aspects. As a result, our organ and immune systems attain optimum functioning; which is the key to good health.

Qigong involves three important aspects: mind, physical movement, and breath. One cannot call an exercise Qigong if the exercise is missing any one of the above. Your mind focuses on your breath and your breath controls your body movements. This kind of practice provides many health benefits.

- Your mind should be calm and completely empty, without any thoughts. This kind of emptiness regulates the neurochemicals in your brain, thus providing harmonious energy flow to the body.
- Your breath should be quiet, deep, and slow, allowing your body to receive more oxygen, which provides fundamental energy.
- Your body movements should be slow. Slow movements work with the breath in a unique way, allowing Qi to flow smoothly in the body.

There are five distinct Qigong traditions: Daoist, Confucian, Buddhist, martial arts, and medical. Chinese medical Qigong is beginning to attract a great deal of attention outside of China. Qigong was suppressed during the Cultural Revolution, but never died out. Today in China, more than 100 million people practice this self-healing exercise on a daily basis. Many people are healed from this ancient healing art, and more and more people around the world are becoming interested in this ancient energy practice. In 1988, the Chinese held the first world conference to highlight Qigong medical research. These conferences have grown in popularity over the past decade and have been held in other countries.

Qigong has a close relationship with Chinese medicine. Qigong is part of the Chinese healing arts; it is a type of disciplined, self-healing therapy. Qigong is considered a form of natural healing, preventive, and longevity medicine. Many people have recovered after suffering long-term illness by using Qigong practice; the resulting improvements, cures, and recoveries were considered miraculous. When I was in medical school, I never believed in Qigong; but now I am teaching and practicing it on a regular basis. Qigong is one of the most powerful prescriptions a TCM doctor can give because it works directly on the body's energy system. This energy system can boost the immune function and balance hormones and other biochemical elements in the body.

> One of my patients had knee surgery. The doctor told him that his healing process was amazing and asked him what he was doing beside regular work. He told the doctor the only difference was that he practiced Qigong regularly.

Qigong is very good at correcting immune system disorders, chronic pain, and other chronic ailments. In China, medical practitioners in hospitals often prescribe Qigong for treating arthritis, asthma, bowel problems, diabetes, migraines, heart disease, hypertension, high stress, anxiety, and many other disorders.

In China, Qigong has also been used to treat cancer, and to reduce the side effects of chemotherapy and radiation therapy. Cancer patients often receive great benefits with Qigong practice; many are even healed with Qigong practice. To many Western medical scientists, using Qigong to treat cancer is thought to be questionable. There is, however, much evidence and testimonials from cancer survivors who have practiced Qigong during their healing process. It cannot be denied that Qigong has prolonged people's lives.

It has been well documented that Qigong practice speeds recovery from surgery and injuries. With Qigong practice, the cells in the body rejuvenate faster, the organs return to normal functioning quicker, the immune system improves more rapidly, and the tissue recovers faster. All these benefits result from the increase in oxygen in the blood that Qigong provides.

Qigong practice is particularly good for healing problems that Western medicine cannot identify. Frequently, these organ functional problems do not show up in scientific tests. In Western medicine, doctors look for abnormal numbers in blood work, overgrown tissue on x-ray films or MRI, and other anomalies in other tests; but they are less likely to pay attention to the energy of the organs, tissues, and the qualities of biochemicals in the body. For instance, you can have the normal amount of white blood cells but still have poor resistance to all kinds of infections from viruses, bacteria, and other microorganisms.

Qigong practice requirements: Qigong practice requires discipline, confidence, and a positive attitude in order to achieve good results. One should practice on a regular basis, not just a short trial to see if it will help. If you have chronic or genetic health issues, it is a lifetime commitment. When you begin to practice, you might not feel the Qi, but after a while, you might feel heat, or tingling, or some kind of strange feeling in your hands or body. You may feel much more relaxed, peaceful, calm, and energetic; your breathing, heart's condition, posture, and outlook toward life all improve. You should avoid negative thoughts when you decide to practice Qigong or use Qigong as part of your life. You must be patient with your progress. If you become frustrated from not seeing any changes within a short period of time, this frustration will let you down. Poor confidence and negative attitude create negative energy, which will interfere with the healing process. The negativity is similar to what happens if you do not like your doctor; you will not follow his or her instructions. You need to practice without any disturbance or interference, and practice without seeking results. Practice faithfully and you will feel the difference within the upcoming year. There are many people who have been disappointed by Qigong's healing, primarily because they did not practice diligently or regularly. Some may have practiced the wrong type of Qigong for their condition.

For more information about Qigong for healing, please refer to my first book *Natural Healing with Qigong*.

In 2001, I took a group of Americans (my students and patients) to China. While there, I injured my leg from overstretching without doing warm-ups first. It was painful and affected my teaching, but I believed it would be better. I continued my exercise and gentle stretching movements I designed for self-therapy. After one year, the pain was completely gone, but you might laugh, "**Only** one year!" A year sounded like a long time, but it was worth every moment to be able to return to normal. For some people, an injury like that could have caused them soreness for a lifetime, but I am now entirely back to normal. I once had a student, a fibromyalgia sufferer, who attended my Therapeutic Qigong workshop. She then purchased the videotape and practiced at home. After four months of daily practice, most of her symptoms were gone. She could not believe this could happen, because she had seen so many doctors and no one could help her.

Taiji (Tai Chi)*

Taijiquan is called Tai Chi Chuan by most Americans. They are the same thing. Taiji (Tai Chi) is another internal energy exercise for strengthening both mind and body. Originally, Taiji was derived

---

* In this book, we use the term Taiji because the earliest Chinese immigrants who came to the U.S. were Cantonese (who spoke a different dialect from Mandarin, the national language); many of the spellings in Pinyin are taken from Cantonese. These different spellings have caused much confusion.

from the martial arts, which was created in late Ming and early Qin Dynasties in a small village in Henan Province in China. Now Taiji has become a way of maintaining good health and longevity. Taiji is a very sophisticated, well-choreographed exercise that involves slow and circular movement, mental concentration, controlled breathing, and a balanced and relaxed posture. Taiji practice harmonizes the body and mind, promotes energy circulation, and builds a strong and well-balanced body.

> I had a student who once told me at the first class of beginning Taiji that it was impossible to learn. I told her not to worry, and promised her that she would learn Taiji well. After 10 classes, she surprised herself because she was able to perform Taiji with a relaxed posture. Not only had she learned the Taiji form, she experienced calmness and felt much more relaxed after suffering from long-term anxiety.

Most Chinese people (in mainland China) practice Taiji for health maintenance, so they do not necessarily study Taiji in depth. These are mostly retired people. A small number of younger people, however, are deeply involved with the fundamentals and essence of Taiji. It is their special passion that motivates them to become masters.

In many situations, Taiji can be used for healing. That Taiji practice improves balance has been documented in a study of 60 patients at Harvard Medical School. Patients were much less wobbly after 10 weeks of Taiji practice. The school also studied Taiji's effects on heart disease. The study involved 30 patients with heart failure who practiced Yang-style Taiji for 12 weeks. The group who practiced Taiji increased its exercise capacity, whereas the control group decreased its capacity. They also found autonomic tone improved for the patients in the Taiji group. In 2008, the Harvard Medical School is using our students to research the effect of Taiji on osteopenia.

Here is good news for those who practice Taiji. In addition to improving balance and coordination, the gentle exercise also seems to increase immunity, particularly to the virus that causes shingles. A study in California, Los Angeles described in the September 2003 issue of *Psychosomatic Medicine* showed that a group of older men and women who took Taiji courses for 45 minutes three days a week showed an increase of up to 50 percent of memory T-cells, immune system cells that recognize and attack the varicella herpes virus that causes shingles. You are vulnerable to shingles if you ever had chickenpox because the virus responsible can remain dormant in nerve cells indefinitely. With age, immunity often weakens, allowing the virus to reactivate. The result is shingles, a disorder that frequently causes blistering on the skin and can be extremely painful.

Taiji can be used for treating mild depression. Using a specific form of Taiji (16-Step Taiji, a medical form for healing) along with specific music, provides immediate results in changing one's mood. This change has happened to many students in my school. For details about using Taiji for healing depression, please refer to my book *Taiji for Depression* (sold at Chinese Medicine for Health, Holliston, MA).

Important tips for practicing Taiji: Practicing Taiji requires patience, full concentration, relaxation, diligent practice, and learning in a non-competitive environment.

The first thing in Taiji practice is to train yourself to be relaxed. If you are not relaxed, you cannot do Taiji well, nor can you receive the benefits. All Taiji movements require relaxation. Your mind has to relax first, and then your body will become relaxed. You constantly train your muscles to let go of tension, your mind to let go of worry and anger. These tensions, worries, and anger can block your energy (Qi) flow in the body. In Chinese medicine, Qi blockages are a large part of poor health. We must let go of our physical and mental tensions, grudges, prejudices, and anything that keeps us tied to the negative past. Doing so allows us to flow more easily into the future by clearing our mind and body of old stress so we can constantly find a fresh perspective on life. If you feel tight in any part of the body, you need to stop and start again, with complete relaxation. Do not be afraid to stop and start again at any time.

When I first took lessons from Master Feng Zhi Qiang (a grandmaster in the Chen-style of Taijiquan) in Beijing during the summer of 2002, all he said to me was "you are too tight, you must relax." I thought I was pretty good, but I decided to try to relax more, and once I started to pay more attention to relaxation, my form and skill in push hands (two-person Taiji practice) and balance improved greatly.

The next thing to develop in Taiji practice is patience. It is a long journey that may take a lifetime. You will not receive the benefits of Taiji if you do not want to invest time to practice. There is no shortcut, no quick way to learn either Taiji or Qigong, but it is a good journey that will give you a lifetime of benefits. You should not be frustrated if you have a problem during your learning journey. In the beginning, you might feel the difficulty as you try to learn the circular and non-stop movements. If you continue to practice, you will feel much more relaxed and comfortable. Once you start to see the improvement in both Taiji practice and your health, you will start to love it and will not want to give it up. If you really want to learn Taiji, you must practice diligently.

Taiji practice requires full concentration. You should leave all thoughts behind; have your mind completely empty. If your mind is not clear, you cannot practice Taiji well. If you think too much during practice, you might make the movements worse. If your mind starts to wander off, you may lose awareness of the energy center. Only with focused practice will you experience the benefits of moving meditation and moving energy. The focus can also help you to find your energy center.

Diligent practice with a non-competitive mind is also very important. One cannot achieve without diligent practice. Both Taiji and Qigong are like energy food that the human body needs. Taiji practice is not for competition. It is for your own well-being, to prevent disease, build inner peace, delay aging, and heal illness. You only compete with yourself time after time, not with other people. If you see that someone is better than you are or who learns the movements more quickly than you, you should not be discouraged.. We are all slow learners in some areas, and may be faster other areas; this is normal. Slow learners can be good, solid learners, and become experts in the future; while quick learners can be superficial learners. The most important thing is to enjoy the practice thoroughly; you will improve week by week, month by month, or year after year.

Taiji promotes internal strength physically, mentally, and emotionally. That strength comes from building strong Qi, which is why it can be a powerful training tool for martial artists. However, you do not have to be a martial artist to benefit from Taiji. People of all ages practice Taiji. Many people with disabilities and ailments also practice Taiji as a therapy. The practice of Taiji is a long, remarkable, and healthy journey. It is a journey to longevity and happiness.

Tips for Practicing Qigong or Taiji

In general, there is no contraindication in Taiji (Tai Chi) and Qigong (Qi Gong) practice. However, these tips will help you to achieve better results.

1. A person who does not believe Qigong can improve health somewhat, but not truly arrive at good results. Just think about when someone tells you what to do. If you do not believe this person, you will not always do what he tells you. If you do not believe that a Japanese car is better than American car, you would prefer to buy an American car. You do what you believe. This is what Chinese medicine says, that the mind controls the body. Your mind, your consciousness, and your beliefs guide your behavior; your behavior in most cases represents who you are. Sometimes when you do not believe something, but are willing to try it, you might change your mind and beliefs because of the positive outcome.

2. Drink water before morning practice. Half a glass of warm water is a mild wake-up call to your organs, especially the stomach. In the morning, all of the organs in the body are low in function, and your stomach energy is weak. Drinking warm water can also benefit stomach function by flushing the old stomach juice. It is considered a form of mild cleansing.

3. Practice should not be interrupted. Once you have started practice, you are actually working on moving and building up the flow of energy (Qi). The moving and building up of the energy requires a certain amount of time to accumulate. If you are interrupted during practice, the Qi that you created or built up will be lost. You have to start again, and this takes more time. A tight schedule will create tension, which is counterproductive. You should set up the time and tell your family or friends not to interrupt you during your practice.

4. Females face towards the south whereas males face towards the north, (a practice that might be related to the magnetic atmosphere on earth). If you do not know which way is south or north, you can choose the direction, which you feel good about. This is called "self-judging the Feng Shui." Sometimes choosing your own direction works even better because it fits your energy.

5. Location: Practicing outdoors in nature is the best; green trees and lawns, flower gardens, water sources (even better with moving water) all conducive to good practice. Anywhere in nature is an excellent place to practice. Best of all, you take in more oxygen, which plays an important role in maintaining organ function.

6. Frequency, time, and duration of practice: It is best to practice every day. If you have time to practice every day, 3 to 5 times a week is good. It is important to practice at a regular time. If you have time in the morning, you should do it every morning, (i.e., not in the morning one day and in the afternoon on other days). The practice time can be adjusted to fit your schedule, either a half hour or one hour, even 15 minutes. What is most important is that you do it regularly.

7. Do not practice if the air in the room is not good. Qigong involves breathing, and if the air in the room is not good, it can affect your lungs, which might trigger asthma or other lung diseases. Bad air will interfere with your energy flow, and distract your mind.

8. Outdoor practice: You should avoid heavy winds, because they distract your mind. They also take away the energy that you have created. A practice session in heavy winds is ineffective, and you do not get good results.

9. Do not retain bowels and urine during practice. This is important because they block internal energy flow, and your practice will not be effective.

10. Do not practice when hungry or overfed. If you are hungry during practice, then your energy will be depleted. You might experience dizziness or headache, or you may feel weak after practice. An overfilled stomach causes blockage in the energy system in your body, and your Qi will not go though the channels. Therefore, your practice will not be successful. You might feel more tired after practice.

You can find other details regarding effective practice in my earlier book, *Natural Healing with Qigong*.

People often have the mistaken idea that Qigong and Taiji are too slow, unexciting, and lack enough physical workout. Others have tried to learn Qigong or Taiji, but they have only learned the movements in the form, not the skill in the form. I can teach you all the movements in one day, but that is not real Taiji or Qigong; it is merely joint and muscle movements. You will not feel the Qi, the most important, invisible substance in our body. Only skillful practice can give you this kind of feeling. No one can learn Taiji in a short time. Every master I met has practiced throughout his or her lifetime. Obtaining Qi is based on how much practice you do. Therefore, Taiji looks like a simple, easy, slow, effortless series of body movements, yet it is a very complex exercise and a high-value energy workout.

Turn on your ignition (power switch): This might be the most difficult thing to do for many people. Even though we understand that Taiji and Qigong provide great health benefits, we oftentimes do not do them. The problem is how to get going. Many obstacles can prevent people from starting. Students frequently tell me, "I have to do it", "I know it is good for me, I am going to do it." This, however, is only still in their mind without action. Very often, people tell themselves they want to start, but never act on their good intentions; others will not practice when they feel tired, are too busy, or have too much going on, etc. All these are just excuses that prevent them from starting. I do not want to say they lack willpower; maybe they lack understanding or patience. As mentioned before, besides providing other benefits, Taiji and Qigong can reduce stress. In modern life, we need these kinds of exercises even more, to balance our lives. With Taiji or Qigong practice, your stress is minimized and allows you to enjoy better health and more peace, and enjoy the money you work hard to earn. Fatigue/tiredness might be a good motivation for practice, because you feel better after practice; feeling stiff should be a good motivation to practice, too. All you have to do is set aside a convenient time and start moving your body within that timeframe. Instead, some people choose to lie on the couch, which makes the feeling of tiredness even more predominant. Students have often told me that they felt tired before class, but that they felt much better after practice. "Too busy" is not a good excuse either; certainly you can spare 15 or 30 minutes out of 24 hours. In some cases, being too busy could damage your health, especially to your heart and brain. You do not realize it until you are older, and then it is sometimes too late.

Turning on your ignition is the key. You just have to do it without hesitation: go to a class or put a Taiji recording into the VCR, follow the beautiful music, and move your body.

Chapter 5

Daoist Healing

Daoism (Taoism) started as a combination of psychology and physiology but evolved into a religious faith in 440 A.D., when it was adopted as a state religion. Daoism, along with Buddhism and Confucianism, became one of the three great religions of China. With the end of the Ching Dynasty in 1911, state support for Daoism ended and much of the Daoist heritage was destroyed during the next period of warlordism. Along with other religions, Daoism was restricted for many years until 1982 when Deng Xiao Ping began to govern China.

Daoism has had a significant impact on North American culture in areas of acupuncture, herbalists, holistic practices, natural healing therapy, and martial arts practice. (See www.religioustolerance.org/Daoism.htm for more detail.)

Dao (Tao) means the Natural Way, following what is most alive and spontaneous. Its guiding principle is to follow what is natural to you, and your own inner nature will unfold effortlessly. Therefore, everyone unfolds differently. The only person you need to follow is yourself; you perform whatever is right for you! Many Buddhists, Christians, and Sufis study Dao, because it helps ground the spirit into the body. The Daoist (Taoist) principles of Qi, the energy or life force that is, Qi) are the same for all creatures. They are based on balancing the receptive and expansive, or Yin and Yang, forces that resonate within every body, every society, and every atom of nature. These pathways have been thoroughly mapped for over thousands of years.

Every occupation, every person can benefit from Daoist practice. You do not have to be sick to learn the Dao. Dao leads you to a relaxed state, which allows you to reach new levels of health. By enhancing your mind's powers, it stops the stresses before they cause physical disorders. It dramatically increases your tolerance level, allowing you to be more effective at what you do, and to live in peace. It can increase your pleasure with almost everything you do. Moreover, it allows your energy channel to open, thereby preventing disease.

Daoist practice can also help enhance creativity. Once you tap into the inner peace of your life, you can channel your newfound wisdom into any area of your life. Let Daoist wisdom guide you. Let the energy unleash your creativity. It will move the artist's brush, write the novel, play the music or sports, and find whatever else you like and enjoy.

No matter how the outside world is, the Daoist still keeps this inner peace; your spirit grows ever stronger. You are guided by trust in your own direct experience.

The Daoist practice creates a positive mind and attitude. You are more apt to accept than fight to win. Many times after practice, you will win without fighting; you will then appreciate the power of the Dao. Daoism teaches one to be grateful for one's life and accept whatever nature provides, which is part of the reason that the Daoist does not hold on to negativity. One of the most important parts of the Daoist practice is to let go and focus on the present, which helps you to be more relaxed, more focused, creative, peaceful, and effective with whatever you are doing, and have more happiness throughout life. Daoism offers tremendous mental benefits, which are most important in maintaining good health and preventing disaster.

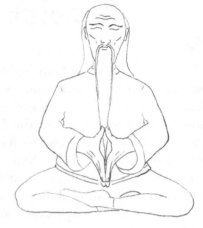

Meditation, part of Daoist practice.

Daoism is not a religion, but can be a religion if you want it to be. Daoism allows people to have faith, religion, or beliefs, as they choose. Daoists accept whatever nature offers. Daoism is a relaxed life practice.

In contrast with Western religion, which considers man as separate from God, the Daoist philosophy sees man and nature as one; man is part of nature. Nature changes in ways similar to the ways a person's body changes. For instance, when the weather changes, people can feel more aches and pains before the storm comes. This is because the body's energy changes too. Nature supplies all sources for humans, and humans find answers from nature for every inquiry.

The study of the Dao is a journey requiring both reading and practice. Studying alone without practice will not give you full benefits. You must apply what you learn in your life. Some of the chapters in *Dao De Jing* (*Tao Te Ching, Classic on the Virtue of the Dao*), the principle book describing the Dao, can be difficult to understand due to the difficulties in the translations and different historical context of over 2,000 years ago. Due to the differences in the cultural background, some information might not be appropriate for modern living, but the Dao still provides valuable information for us. It is a treasure from our Chinese ancestors. We can just take from it whatever information is suitable to us to help our life and mental health.

Steps in learning the Dao involve:
1. Reading the *Dao De Jing* is the first step. You do not have to put much pressure on yourself; just read for fun. You can read either one or two chapters per night, which I prefer or read the whole book at once as you wish.

2. Write down your thoughts that are related to your life after reading each chapter. For instance after reading Chapter 9 Avoiding Excess:

> Better to stop in time than to overfill a vessel.
> Over sharpen a blade and it will soon lose its edge.
> A store of gold and jade cannot be protected.
> Pride in wealth and rank brings calamity on oneself.
> Withdraw when the work is done.
> This is the Dao of heaven.

Write it down if you think it is good, why it is good, and how it can help you. If you think it is not good, or not right, you should write down what part you think is not good or why it is not right. Daoism is not for everyone. What I think is right might not be right for another person. If you are able to write your thoughts down, you can clarify your thinking. Surprisingly, most of my Chinese friends are not Daoist. This is fine; the Daoist accepts everyone.

3. Practice letting go. To practice letting go is also to practice focusing on the present. Only if you can let go of the past, are you able to focus on the present. This is easier said than done. So, constantly tell yourself to let go of the things that bother you, and whatever is not natural for you. The Daoist practice often differs from the Western practice. Western psychotherapy encourages you to talk out your feelings, fears, and past, or whatever is on your mind. It is helpful to give people the chance to let things come out, but it is not helping them let go. After a while, some people just give up going for counseling. Every time you talk about the things that bother you from the past, you re-imprint these negative images onto your mind, and reinforce the negative memory. Some people can never let go. The Daoist practice wants you to forget

Daoist study has changed my life by making it much more relaxed. Before I started on the Daoist path, my stress level was extremely high. I did not know how to deal with stress in a natural way. During the Chinese Cultural Revolution (1966-1976), there was much chaos within families and the country itself. I was very frustrated because I could not do what I wanted to do. Because I was not able to express myself, internal stagnation caused energy blockages and physical problems within me. Daoist study and practice over these years has helped me to change my attitude, lifestyle, diet, health, work, relationships, learning expectations, and so on. I came to realize this because the closer I am to nature, the more relaxed I am; the more relaxed I am, the easier my life is; the easier my life is, the happier I am; the happier I am, the better everything comes together.

about the things in the past that were unpleasant, so you can move on to a new day, a new life, a better life. Daoist therapy will ask you to say every morning, "from now on, I will…"; "today, I will…"

4. Making decisions. Before making a decision, ask yourself if this step is natural or not natural? Is this right to me or not right to me? If you feel this decision is not natural, not really right, you need to reconsider, unless you are obligated. Only the natural feeling is with the Dao.

5. Try to be with nature as often as you can. The more you are with nature, the more you feel the Dao. Besides, outdoor activities provide more oxygen, which is very important to keep us healthy.

6. Practice Yin and Yang. Everything has two sides — the positive and the negative. Nothing is perfect. If you are looking for a perfect place, or a perfect person to be your life partner, perfect child, perfect house to buy, you are going against the Dao. You just have to look into the positive side of things if the negative side does not bother you too much. If the thing is much more negative than positive, you know it is not the right thing for you, so you might like to change it.

7. Practice Taiji (Tai Chi) and Qigong regularly. Both originated from the Daoist practice; the movements are spontaneous and natural. This kind of practice helps you develop the natural flow of energy within you, which automatically allows you to let go and move on.

Chapter 6

Cancer Prevention and Healing

Cancer is a very difficult topic to write about. People often ask if there is proof that Chinese medicine and exercise actually works. How can you guarantee this will work? This doubt often prevents people from trying new things. They would rather go through traditional therapies such as chemotherapy and radiation therapy. People frequently die, not from cancer, but from infection due to the weakened immune system that results from the body losing its fight against cancer. If you do not try some other way, how do you know other things will not work? At least try these new approaches.

For centuries, people thought cancer was impossible to prevent and impossible to heal. Even in modern society, with modern medicine, cancer is still a focal point for medical people to explore the cause and the cure. Much research has been done with Western medicine using drug therapy, but there has not been enough research into Eastern medicine and natural approaches. People with cancer have been cured from different natural methods but there is no evidence to prove how they were cured. Cancer patients lived much longer than the doctors had expected, but how? Nobody could put the "how" on paper in a convincing way. This is the frustration of Chinese medical doctors who know that there are natural ways of healing cancer and they work. Because there is a lack of research based on evidence except for individual cancer patients' positive experience with natural medicine, it is difficult for Chinese medicine practitioners to educate people about these natural ways. As a doctor of Chinese medicine, as a healer, and as an educator, I think it is important to communicate information about cancer prevention that has been collected from my lifetime of healing experience. As a Western-trained medical practitioner who also practices Chinese medicine, I intend to present the different views of two kinds of healing systems (Eastern and Western), and relay life experiences collected from cancer survivors.

First, I think that cancer itself is not terrible; the terrible part is the mind and the stagnated Qi. Cancer is curable if the mind is healthy and the Qi is flowing smoothly in the body. In contrast, cancer cannot be cured if your mind is not healthy, or if your Qi is blocked or weak. A healthy mind does not mean you must be stubborn, and strong Qi does not mean you need to have big muscles in your body. A healthy mind helps to promote Qi flow, and smoothly flowing Qi helps to create a positive and peaceful mind.

What Causes Cancer?

We often think that cancer could be caused by certain chemicals, high power electric fields, certain fungus or mold, a certain bacteria or virus, and so on. Nevertheless, even when we are exposed to these pathogens all the time, why do some people get cancer and others do not. In Chinese medicine, things are viewed differently. As we know, cancer tissue (tumor) is a very hard object; almost like a stone that the doctor has to remove surgically. How does the normal tissue grow like a stone? From many years of clinical experience with Chinese medicine, TCM doctors realize that after the body has stored the stagnated Qi for a long time and it has not been corrected, blood stagnation occurs. These stagnations cause weakness in the immune system and certain tissues are undernourished. Therefore, the normal tissue becomes cancerous tissue. People who have better immune function can fight the cancer with other treatments, such as chemotherapy, radiation, or Chinese medicine. If the immune function is weak, a person with cancer might lose the ability to fight and die in the end. Many things can cause stagnation of the Qi, such as high stress, wrong diet, low mental tolerance, an inactive lifestyle, mental restrictions, overworked body and mind, excessive drinking, smoking, certain uncorrected injuries, long-term depression, an introverted personality, other illnesses not corrected in a timely manner, etc. Even the pathogens mentioned earlier could cause stagnation of Qi and blood.

Early Prevention

From early childhood, we need to create a peaceful and healthful environment. This does not mean you have to give a child whatever it wants. A healthy environment includes constantly teaching which behaviors are the right things to do is and which to avoid; what the right food to eat is and what the food to avoid is. Children might not listen now, but after they hear the message so many times, these words do start to sink in. When I was young, my mother used to tell me which food had good nutrition and which food did not, when I was young. It is not easy for some parents, and might be a constant battle, but these efforts will prevent more serious health problems in the future. If the parents do not know what is right and wrong, the kids will not learn to make the right choices as they grow. We always think we know how to raise our kids, but in many cases, we do not and we make mistakes. When we realize we have made a mistake, we sometimes say to ourselves, "I wish I could do this over" or "if I could go back in time, I would do it differently." Educating parents is just as important as educating children. With appropriate care and teaching by the parents, children grow up with a better understanding of life and health, and they cope better with stress. This is part of preventing cancer, because the unmanaged stress stored in the body can cause stagnation of Qi, and the stagnation of Qi can cause cancer. Upon reviewing the cases of my cancer patients, I find that almost every one of them had drastic stress in their lives. People often ask me why they got cancer with no history of cancer in their family. It is useless to discuss with them the question of "why," for the damage is done, and knowing why cannot turn back time. Instead, they need to understand the healing path and lifestyle changes they need to make to go forward. Moreover, people who do not have cancer need to know how to prevent it.

The next section provides you with tips for healthful living and healing.

Tips for Preventing Cancer

1. Do not let the stress in your daily life go on too long; it can do much damage later. As we now know that stresses causes Qi stagnation. We also know that stagnated Qi can cause cell mutation or tumors to grow.
2. Create smooth Qi; take care of body disharmony or imbalance early. Do not let discomfort stay with you for too long. Some minor discomfort could be the beginning stages of cancer.
3. Develop healthy habits, such as a moderate lifestyle, healthy diet, regular exercise, avoid too much smoking and drinking, and so on.
4. Avoid using various chemicals for a long time.
5. Stay with the Dao.
6. Keep a positive outlook and attitude as much as you can, which is influential in preventing cancer.
7. Laugh and joke more. Laughing is an excellent healing methodology. When you lose the ability to laugh, you lose a big part of your life. Laughing can also prevent depression, which could cause cancer.
8. Do more outdoor activities.

Tips for Natural Healing

1. Maintain a balanced stomach function, stay on a vegetarian diet. (See the many recipes at the end of this book.)
2. Build a healthy mind; do not let anything interfere with your healing.
3. Deal with depression as soon as possible; reduce stress as soon as possible. (See the section on Daoism.)
4. Avoid using alcohol; avoid smoking, chemicals, and other pathogenic substances.
5. Get as much fresh air as possible.

6. Do cancer-healing exercises daily, as described below.
7. Drink more water; listen to your body, which sometimes tells you that it needs water.
8. Pay attention to all of the items in "Tips for Preventing Cancer," described above.
9. Take Chinese tonic herbs to boost your immune system, as well as regular Chinese medical therapy, such as acupuncture, Chinese massage, Chinese exercise, and so on.
10. Avoid overuse of the body.

A Chinese woman who lived in Canada suffered from cancer, and the doctor gave her two weeks to live. But she recovered, which surprised everyone, including her doctor. Part of her success was her diligent practice of Chinese exercise, Tai Chi, Qigong, and martial arts. I have heard so many stories that people who had cancer healed from regular exercise. In fact, one of my students told me his martial art teacher has been cancer free for the past 20 years.

Exercise Routines for Healing Cancer

Cancer-healing exercises are designed to boost the immune system, improve energy and blood circulation, bring about organ harmony and speed up the healing process. In many cases, your own immune system will fight the cancer for you. Many people who have cancer do not realize the importance of exercise as a part of healing, and they often wait to do it until the final stages of cancer, when it is too late. Once you have cancer, it does not matter which kind, you need to practice every day no matter what. Sometimes you do not want to practice because you are tired, but you will feel that you have more energy once you finish these exercises. The miracle is in your hands, and you can make it happen.

Make a plan for your routine:

1. Walk 20 minutes. First, walk at a moderate speed for 5 minutes, then fast for another 10 minutes, finally slowing it for the last 5 minutes. This kind of walking is intended to get your blood circulation moving.
2. Do special cancer-healing Qigong (Open Channel Qigong) for 10 to 15 minutes. (See the appropriate section in this chapter for further details.) This workout allows you to relax your whole body, strengthen your muscles, release tension, open the channels, and minimize aches and pain in your body. Stretching can be individualized according to your specific tightness or problems.
3. Go through Eight Brocade Qigong (Ba Duan Jing). This particular Qigong enhances your immune system and increases your energy level. (See the

appropriate section in this chapter for further details.) Alternate this exercise with the 16-step Taiji form. An instructional DVD on this form of Taiji is available from the New England School of Tai Chi and Qi Gong.

4. Practice the 16-Step Taiji form (a medical form of Taiji for healing) two times continuously (this will take about 12 minutes total). This form of Taiji balances the internal organs and brings back the harmony between mind and body, which in turn improves the immune system and promotes healing. Alternate this exercise with the Eight Brocade Qigong (Ba Duan Jing).

5. Drink a glass of warm water after the exercise, which helps to cleanse the body.

Qigong Exercises for Healing Breast Cancer

This sequence of Qigong exercises not only helps to open the meridian system, but also helps to enhance the immune system, which is the key to fighting cancer, and promotes healing.

The entire group of cancer healing exercises only takes less than an hour. If you spend time every day for three months, you will likely see a big difference in all aspects of your health. Even doing these exercises just three or four times a week would be still very helpful in improving the immune function, which helps to fight cancer. It is worthwhile to explore these exercises. Once you feel better, you will be encouraged and want to exercise regularly. Nevertheless, even after you start to feel better, it does not mean you can stop; you need to continue these exercises to prevent a relapse and maintain optimum health. Once you establish a routine, you might not want to stop; because you feel good, you might develop a positive "addiction" to regular exercise.

Qigong Warm-Up Exercises

1. Turn body from side to side. Feet are placed shoulder width apart with arms raised to a comfortable height, turn body from side to side. Repeat 1 to 2 minutes.

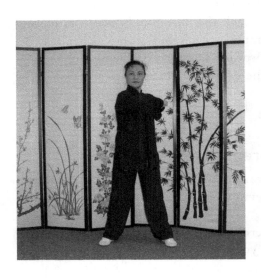
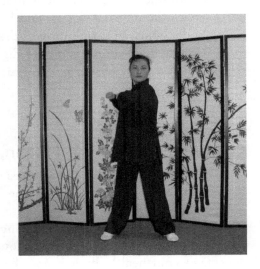

2. Push and pull with steady pace. Feet are placed shoulder width apart, push right hand forward and left hand, palm facing up at waist level; push left hand forward and right hand palm facing up at waist level.

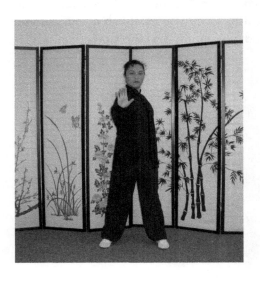
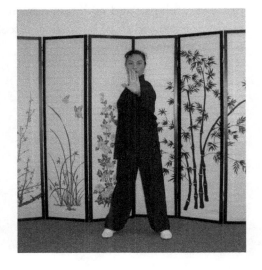

3. Move shoulders up and down, roll forward / backward, alternate roll forward / backward.

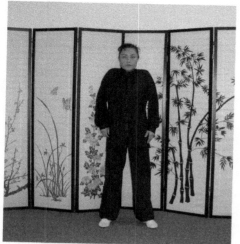
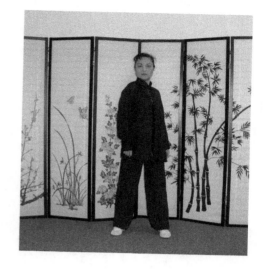

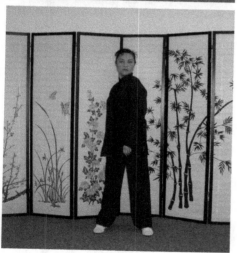

4. Slowly move head in all directions; to the right, and to the left. Repeat 4 to 8 times. Then move the head up and down 4 to 8 times. Finally move head down from left to right and slowly raise head from left to right.

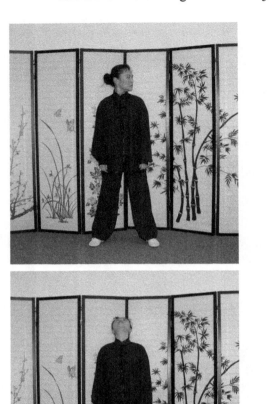
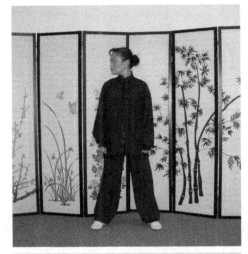
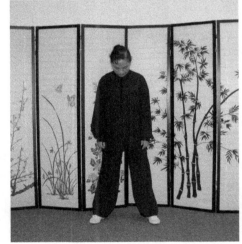

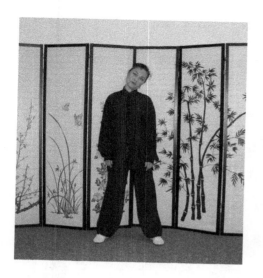

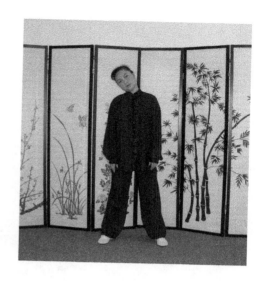

5. Rotate hips with bent knees.

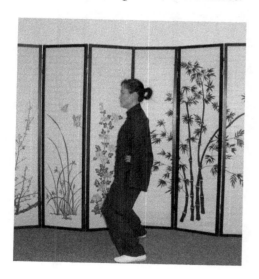

6. Wave body side to side.

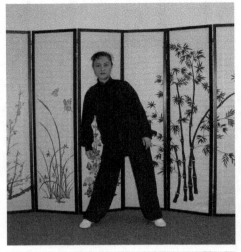
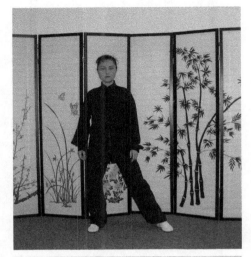
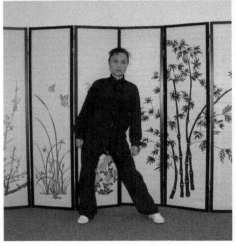
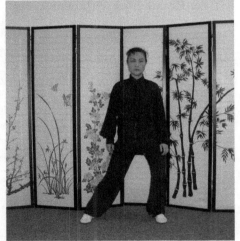

7. Wave body front to back.

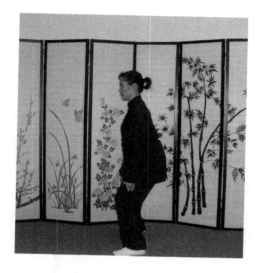 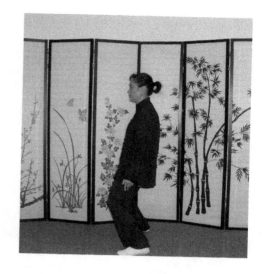

8. Lift and rotate knees.
9. Alternately, circle knees.

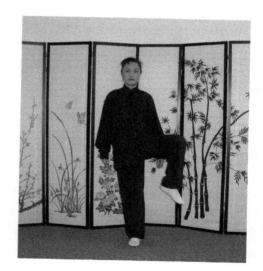

10. Shift weight from left to right while in horse stance. (Horse stance: bend both legs keeping back straight and relaxed.*)

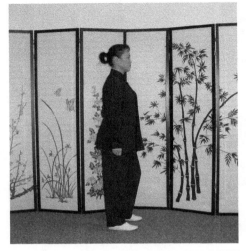
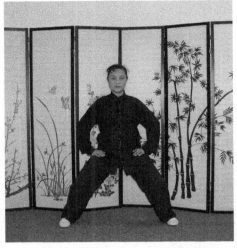
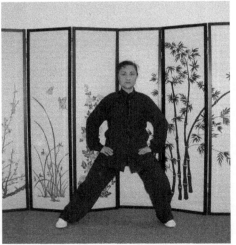
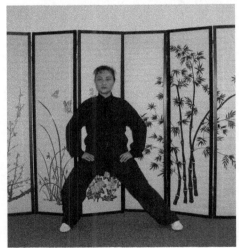

---

* Alternate with bending the knees more with bending lightly. If you have knee problems, bend only slightly.

11. Move up and down while in horse stance.

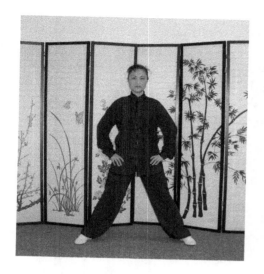 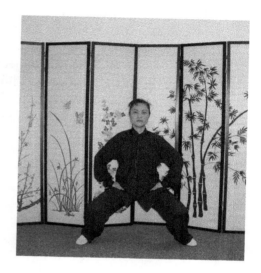

12. Turn body side-to-side while in horse stance.

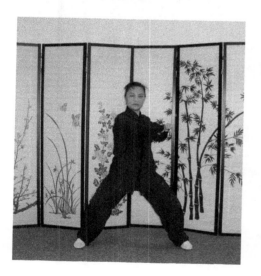 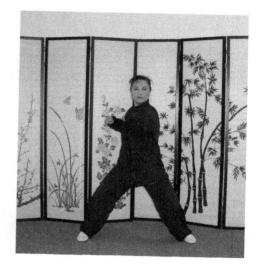

Open Channel Qigong

1. Lifting Qi (Yoga pose):

  a. Facing south, feet spread out to shoulder width. Arms straight out at shoulder level. Palms facing down.

  b. Take a deep breath, simultaneously raise arms and palms together above head, lift as high as you can (lifting the body, too).

  c. While exhaling, bring arms back to shoulder level to beginning stance.

  d. On the fourth time, bring arms all the way down and relax the whole body.

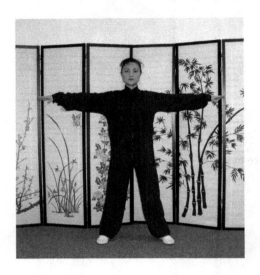 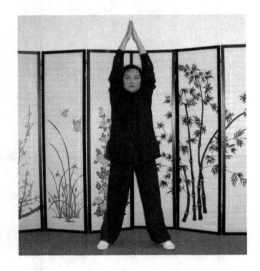

2. Nourish Heart and Kidney (turn body, roll body):

a. Arms straight out at shoulder level; feet spread out at twice the shoulder width.

b. Turn body 90 degrees to left, put weight on right foot with right arm bent.

c. Place right hand in front of your heart (palm facing heart).

d. Place left hand on lower back area (palm facing kidney).

e. Roll body (spin), putting weight to center.

f. Turn body back to starting position and bring arms back to shoulder level

Opposite side:

a. Turn body 90 degrees to right, put weight on left foot with the left arm bent.

b. Place left hand in front of your heart (palm facing heart).

c. Place right hand on lower back area (palm facing kidney).

d. Put weight from left roll to center.

e. Turn body back to starting position and bring arms back to shoulder level.

f. Repeat the movements for each side.

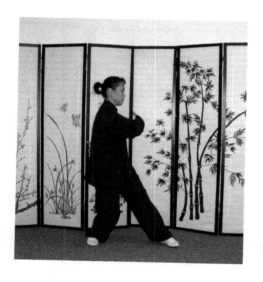 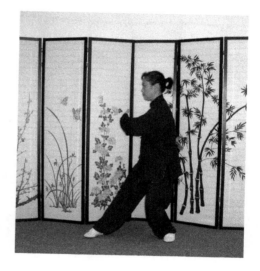

3. Open Liver Channel (bend body to the side, alternate with body rotation):

a. Place feet shoulder width apart.

b. Bend body to the left; at same time, raise right arm straight up above your head along the body to the left; your left arm is next to your left leg, fingers pointing down.

c. The breath is one cycle (inhale then exhale).

d. Bring body upright, slowly bring right arm down; this is also a one-breath cycle (inhale then exhale).

e. Side-bend body to right; at same time, raise left arm straight up above your head along the body to the right; your right arm is next to your right leg, fingers pointing down.

f. The breath is one cycle (inhale then exhale).

g. Bring body upright, slowly bring right arm down; this is also one-breath cycle (inhale then exhale).

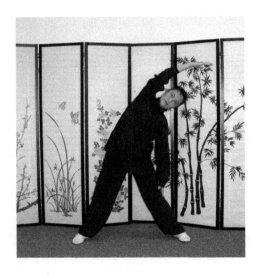 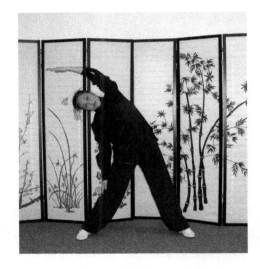

4. Open Kidney and Stomach Channel (bend body forward, touch floor):

a. Feet together, raise hands from front to above head, arms straight (palms facing front).

b. Slowly bend forward, all the way to the floor.

c. Let upper body completely relax for three full breaths.

d. Lower your hips into squatting position and hug knees for three full breaths. Try to keep the heels on the floor.

e. Raise hips slowly with the head hanging down.

f. Slowly roll upper body (spine) up and bring to upright position.

g. Repeat 3 times.

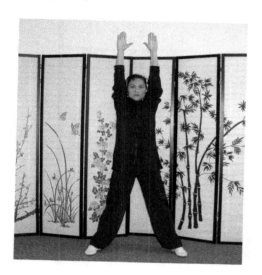 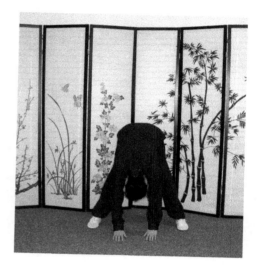

5. Open Lung Channel (Open and close arms):

a. Arms and hands open and close in the front of the chest, combined with breathing.

b. Place hands in front of abdomen as if holding a big ball.

c. Take a deep breath as you bring hands to of the body and squeeze shoulder blades.

d. Exhale and bring hands back to original place as if holding a ball in the front of your abdomen.

e. Open shoulder blades.

f. Repeat 4 times. Breathe deeply and slowly.

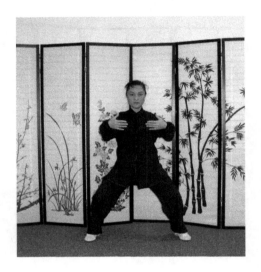 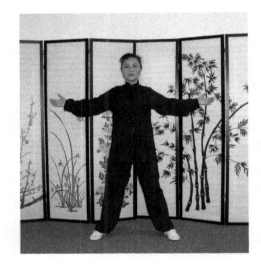

6. Open Spleen Channel (rock the baby, shifting/turning):

a. Place hands in front of your lower abdomen with palms facing up.

b. Turn body and shift weight to left, and start lifting hands up to neck level.

c. Turn body and shift weight to right, as you circle hands to right, then down (keeping hips still).

d. Continue this motion 4 times.

e. Changing sides, circle to opposite side 4 times.

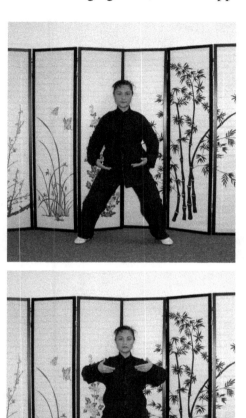
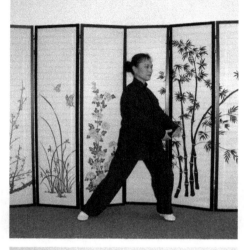
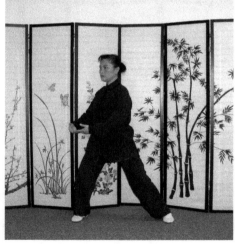

7. Open Upper Dan Tian (Raise hands/arms, turn body):

  a. Place feet shoulder width apart or wider.

  b. Raise arms along side of body, overhead with arms straight; inhale.

  c. Exhale, turn body to left, lowering arms to shoulder level.

  d. Turn body to front, raise arms over your head with arms straight; inhale.

  e. Exhale, turn body to right lowering arms to shoulder level.

  f. Repeat 4 to 8 times.

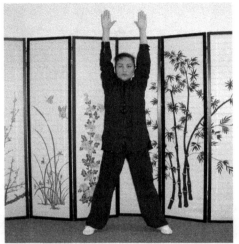
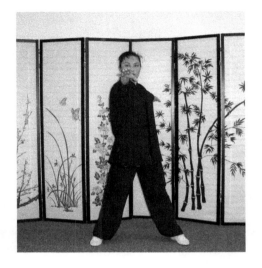
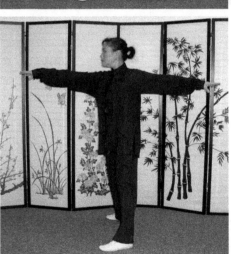

8. Strengthen/Open All Channels (pick up the rock):

a. Stand with feet shoulder width apart.

b. Take a deep breath and raise arms and hands up from front of the body until they extended all the way up.

c. Breathe out and move arms and hands out to side of the body as you start to bend legs without stressing your body.

d. Straighten legs; as you draw in the hands to the center so you feel as if you are picking up a big rock.

e. As you raise your body, allow hands to move along inside of legs, and then up along the body while inhaling.

f. Bring hands and palms down to front as if gently pushing down.

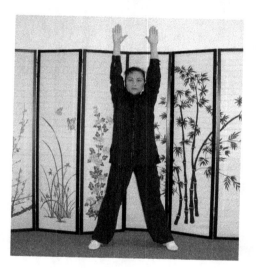
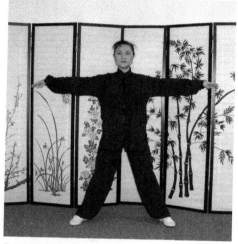
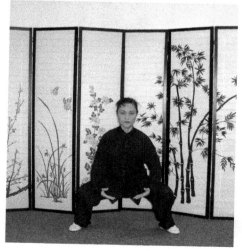

End with deep breath: Raise hands and arms along sides of body; reach all the way up above the head, and slowly press down in front of your body. Repeat 3 times.

Put feet together and relax your whole body.

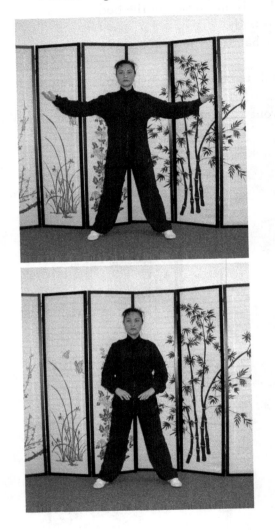
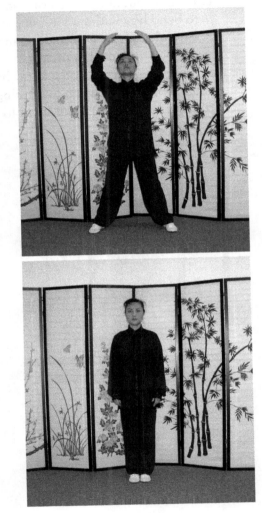

Eight Brocade Qigong (Ba Duan Jing)

Ba Duan Jing Qigong was one of the earliest Qigong forms originating in China. Many other exercises and Qigong forms developed afterwards, based on this group of exercises. The highlight of this group of Qigong is the strengthening of all organs, which provides great benefits in fighting cancer.

1. **Holding Sky Soothing Triple Burner (Shuang Shou Tuo Tian Li San Jiao):**
   a. Feet together, head and body upright, shoulders relaxed; breath evenly, mind focused.
   b. Step out to left, one and a half shoulder width.
   c. Hands in front of the body, overlapping; take a deep breath, raise hands overhead.
   d. Exhale, bring arms to side at shoulder level.

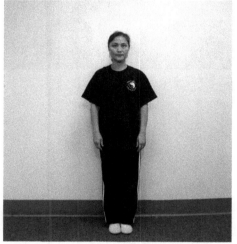
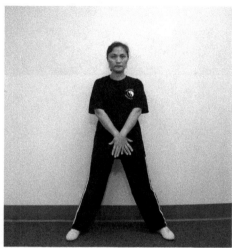
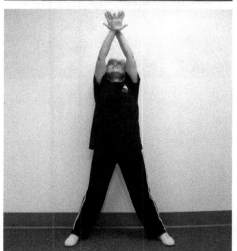
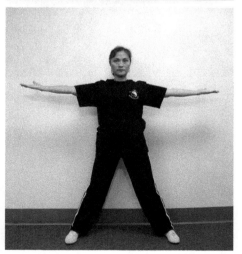

e. Inhale, bend body forward.

f. Exhale, continue bending body downward, hands crossed.

g. Inhale, raise body and hands, push upward above head.

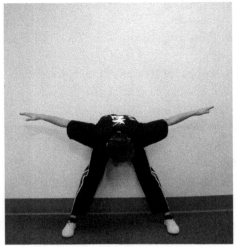
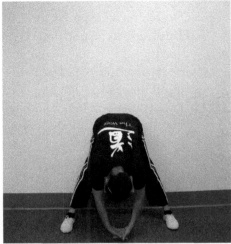
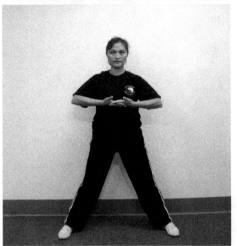
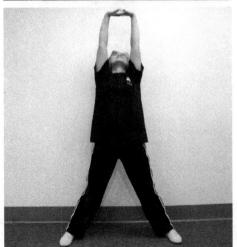

h. Exhale, separate hands to side and relax arms; move hands down next to body.

i. Repeat 4 times.

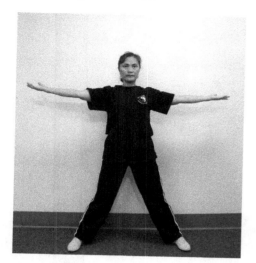
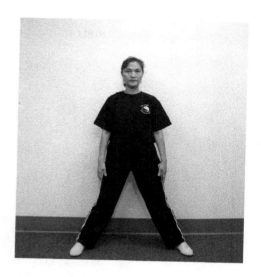

2. Left and Right Shooting the Birds (Zuo Yo Kai Gong She Da Diao):

a. Continue from first movement with feet open.

b. Inhale, arms to side.

c. Exhale, sink body to horse stance, hands crossed in the front of chest.

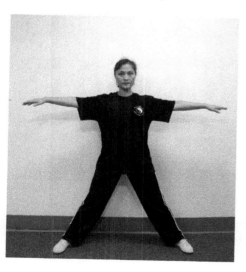
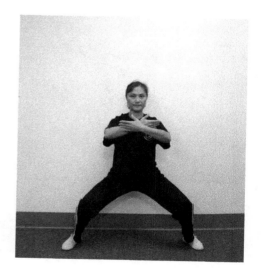

d. Inhale, hands change to fists, then stretch out to side.
e. Exhale, open left hand (only forefinger is straight), push left hand to left at shoulder level.
f. Inhale, open arms to side.
g. Exhale, cross hands in front of your chest.

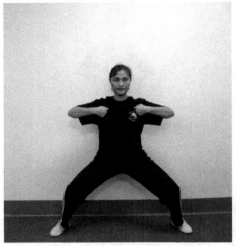

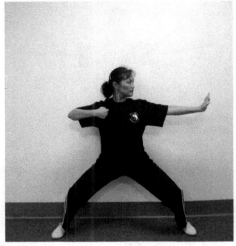

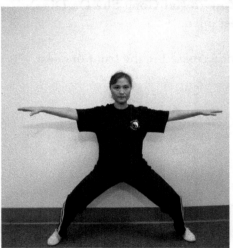

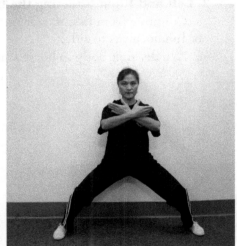

h. Inhale, hands change to fist, then stretch to side.

i. Exhale, open right hand (only forefinger is straight); push right hand to right at shoulder level.

j. Inhale, open arms to side.

k. Repeat above.

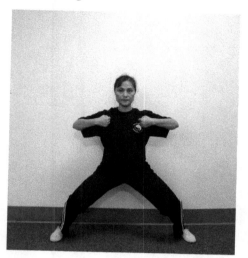 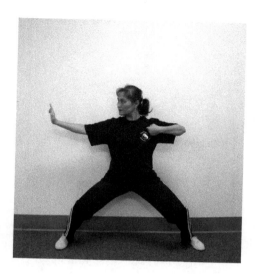

3. Regulate Spleen and Stomach Meridian (Tiao Li Pi Wei Xiu Dan Ju):

a. Step out to left, make fist and open arms to sides.

b. Shift weight to left, turn body to left, move right fist to front at nose level, eyes looking at right fist; left fist is on left waist.

c. Lean body forward, change right fist to open palm and press downward.

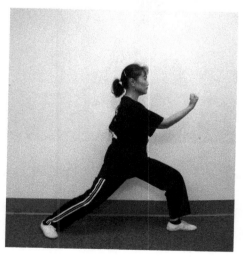 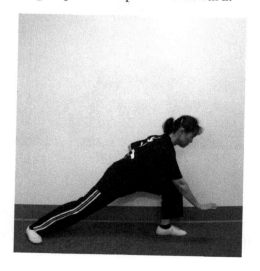

d. Shift weight to right, turn body to right, move right palm (slightly above floor) to right.

e. Turn right palm upward and push up above head, arm straight; left palm pressed down.

f. Change right palm to fist and move down to waist; change left palm to fist and move to front of head at nose level.

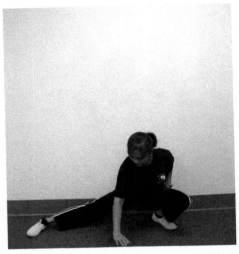
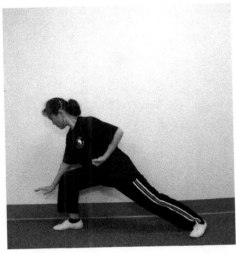
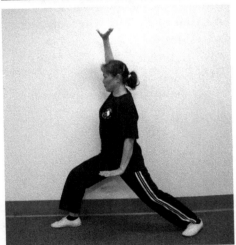
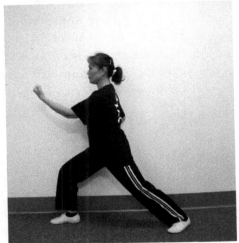

g. Lean body forward; change left fist to palm and press downward.
h. Shift weight to left and turn to left; move left palm (slightly above floor) to left.
i. Turn left palm upward and push up above head, arm straight; right palm pressed down.
j. Repeat above.

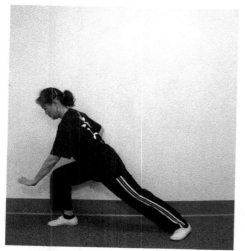
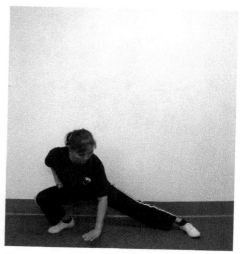
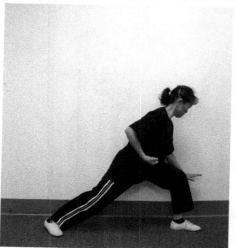
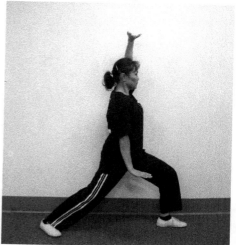

4. Five Burden Seven Disturbance Leave Behind (Wu Lao Qi Shang Wang Hou Qiao):

a. Put weight on right foot, open arms to side, inhale.

b. Step forward with left foot, move hands and arms forward, exhale.

c. Shift weight back, cross hands, inhale.

d. Shift weight to left foot, turn body to left, open arms.

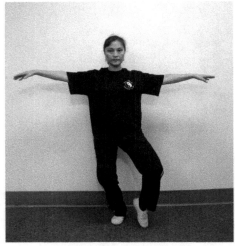 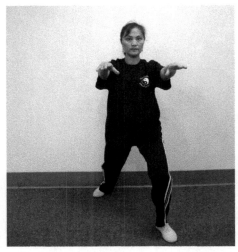

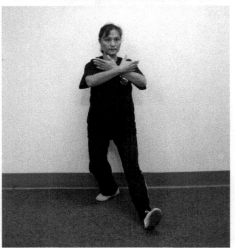 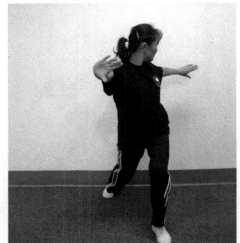

e. Turn body to front, shift weight back, arms crossed.
f. Bring left foot back, hands pressed down.
g. Put weight on left foot, open arms to side, inhale.

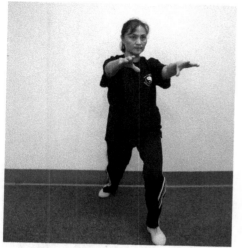
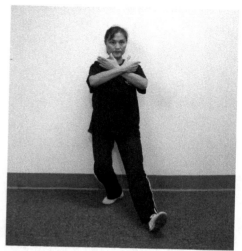
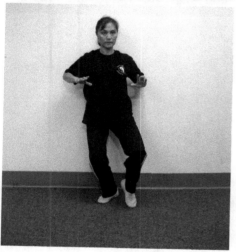
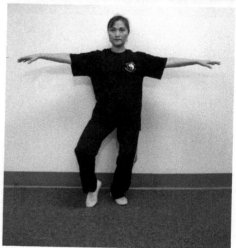

h. Step forward with right foot, move hands and arms forward, exhale.
i. Shift weight back, cross hands, inhale.
j. Shift weight to right foot, turn body to right, open arms.
k. Turn body to front, shift weight back, arms crossed.

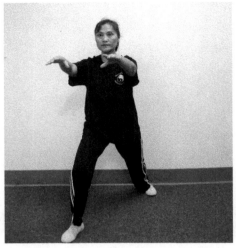
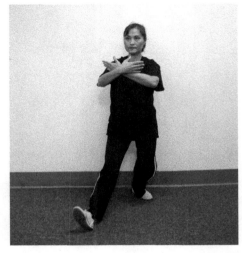
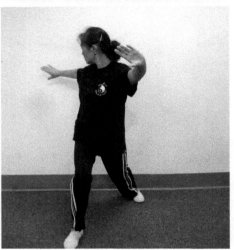
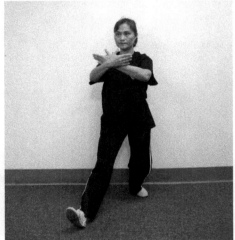

l. Bring right foot back, hands pressed down.

m. Repeat above.

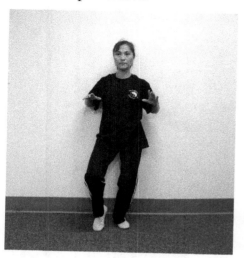
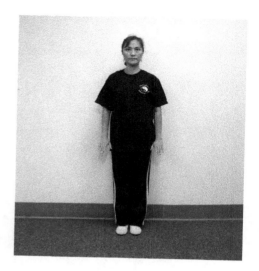

5. Turn Head and Tail Relieve Heart Fire (Yao Tong Bai Wei Qiu Xing Huo):

a. Big step to left.

b. Circle hands up from side of the body, then place hands on your lap, bend both legs (horse stance).

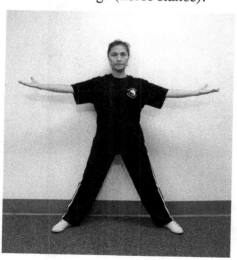
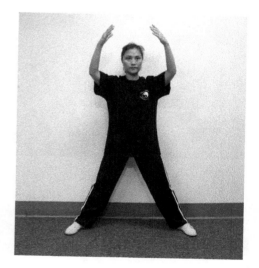

c. Lean body to right/forward.
d. Move body from right to left, eyes looking to right floor
e. Lean body to left/forward.

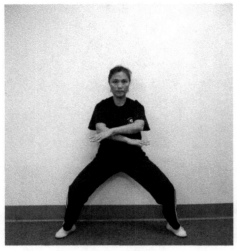
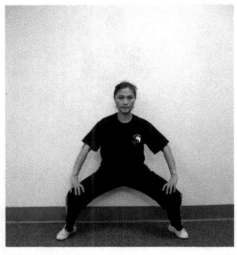
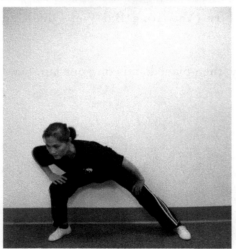
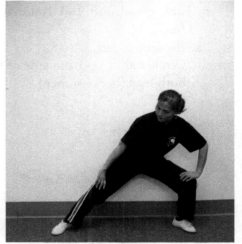

f. Move body from left to right, eyes looking to left floor.
g. Repeat above.

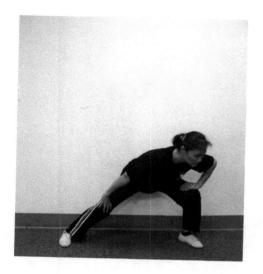
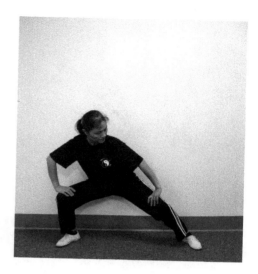

6. Hands Reach Feet Strengthen Kidney and Back (Shuang Shou Pan Zu Gu Shen Yao):
   a. Feet together.
   b. Hands from front of the body move up above head, palms facing front.

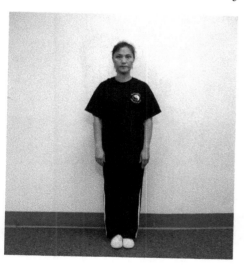
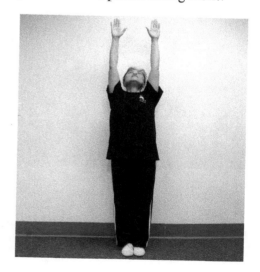

c. Move forward twice in a waving motion from your waist.

d. Bending forward, pinch big toes with hands.

e. Move hands to side, then place behind ankles, slowly move up, over the kidney point.

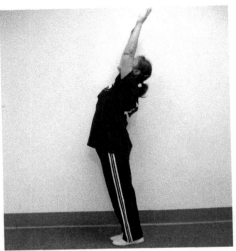

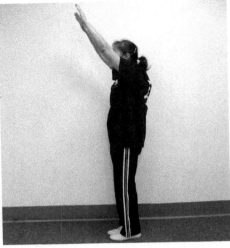

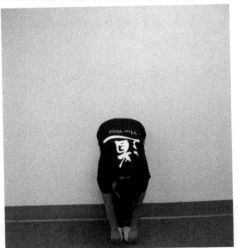

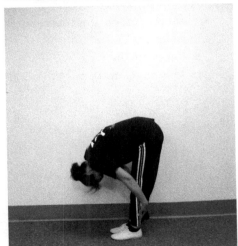

f. Bend backwards, legs straight, hands on kidney point.

g. Straighten body, inhale lifting heels; exhale, move hands down and relax body.

h. Repeat above.

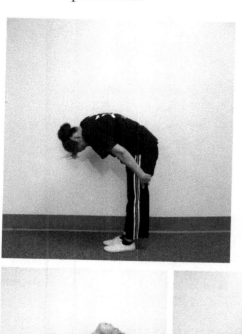
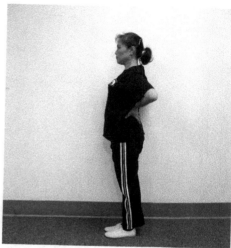
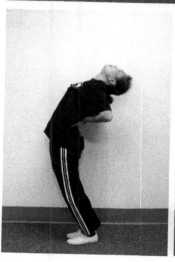
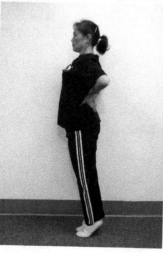
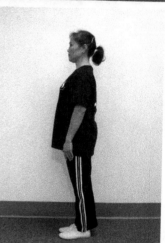

7. Holding Fist Gain Strength (Zua Quan Nu Mu Zheng Li Qi):

a. Big step to left, move hands from front to waist and make a fist, horse stance.

b. Lift right fist, then punch forward; place hand back on waist.

c. Lift left fist, then punch forward; place hand back on waist.

d. Cross hands in the front of the lower abdomen.

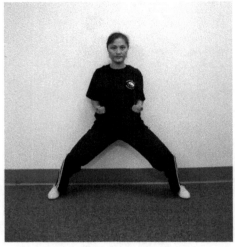
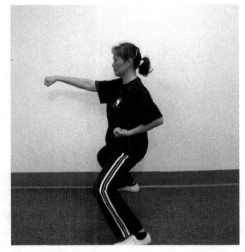
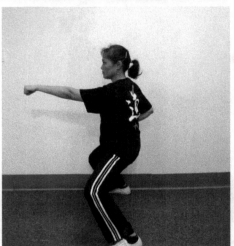
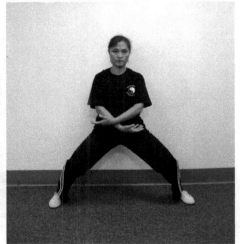

e. Shift weight and turn body to left;, hands circle up above head, then punch down at shoulder level.

f. Move hands to front of the lower abdomen.

g. Shift weight and turn body to right; hands circle up above head, then punch down at should level.

h. Move hands to front of the chest.

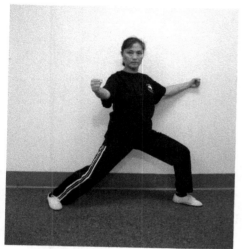
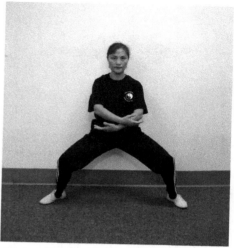
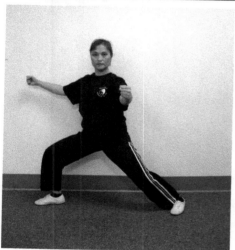
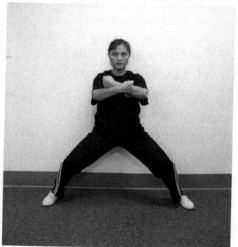

i. Open arms punch to side at shoulder level.

j. Repeat above.

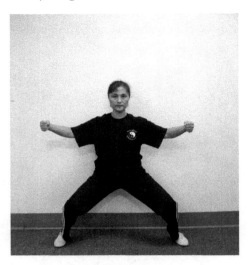

8. Shake Body Eliminate Illness (Bei Hou Qi Dian Bai Bing Xiao):
  a. Feet together.
  b. Move hands on kidney point.
  c. Inhale lifting heels.
  d. Exhale shaking the whole body.
  e. Inhale lifting heels.
  f. Exhale shaking the whole body.
  g. Repeat above.

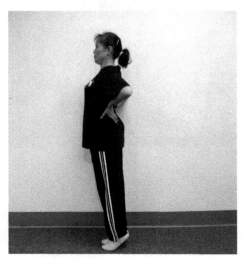

Ending

Take 3 deep breaths, circle arms inward, then place hands over lower abdomen for a minute. Relax whole body.

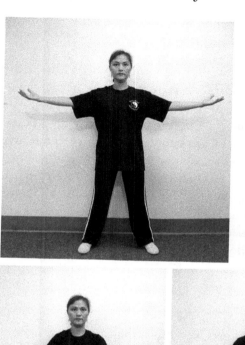
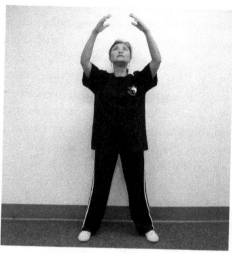
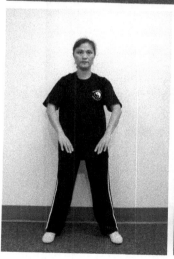
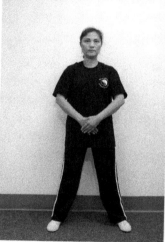
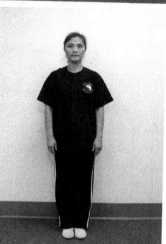

Chinese Herbs for Healing Cancer

Using Chinese herbal medicine to boost the immune system is a common treatment for cancer patients in China. Most Chinese herbal medicines, whether used in a single or combined formula, are tonic immune stimulants. They stimulate blood flow or microcirculation, enhance phagocytosis in the reticuloendothelial system, and affect metabolism and endocrine system.

Many Chinese herbs play an important role in promoting homeostasis in the body. Research has shown that polysaccharide fractions from Chinese herbal medicine have interferon-inducing, anti-tumor, and anti-inflammatory activity, etc.

The majority of cancer patients in China use Chinese herbal medicine in conjunction with chemotherapy or radiation; there are cancer patients prefer to use only herbs. Some herbs that the Chinese medical doctor might use include *Astragalus* (Huang Qi), *Codonopsis pliloulae* (pilose asiabell root), ginseng (Ren Shen), and licorice (Gan Cao). It is important to know that your Chinese medical doctor may use many of these herbs and possibly many others. The TCM doctor will use a specific combination of herbs to treat the specific condition of a certain individual, so you must consult your Chinese medical doctor for individualized treatment.

One cancer patient had been seeing me for two years. Looking at him, you would not know he had cancer. He looked perfectly normal and did not feel sick. His blood test was nearly normal. I knew him well, he could not tolerate any kind of sickness because he so enjoyed being active. Doctors told him that he had only three years to live, unless he underwent a very invasive treatment. This would involve feeling very fatigued, low immune function, nausea and vomiting, sleeping disorder, and side effects that were unpleasant. Afterwards, he would probably experience lifelong side effects. Even with all of these, the success rate was still only 50 percent. This information made him feel sick and he had great deal of anxiety. He was very hesitant and asked my advice regarding his healing path. I told him it was his choice, but I asked him this question: Do you want a quality life for three years or a miserable life for 10 years? He immediately answered that he wanted a quality life for three years, he was not afraid of death. Once he knew what he wanted, he was immediately relieved. I knew he was going to live more than three years, because he allowed his mind to relax, his body to function and the energy to flow smoothly; the channels would be opened. He now still comes to visit me occasionally with full energy and fun. He eats and exercises well, and enjoys the work he does. The one thing that bothers him most is that he does not understand why his cancer specialist did not give him any dietary advice. Instead, the doctor told him he could eat anything he wanted, but he and I both knew that was not the right advice for healing.

Acupuncture for Healing Cancer

Using acupuncture to treat cancer can be very beneficial. Acupuncture not only boosts the immune system, but also balances organ energy. Once organ energy is balanced, the body's healing ability improves. Skilled acupuncturists will often make a plan for a patient's cancer treatment; they will tell you when to start the treatment and when to take a break. Sometimes they will give patients diet suggestions. With treatment, you will experience fewer side effects from chemotherapy and radiation therapy, less fatigue, and better able to maintain daily function. Treatment also helps you to maintain a positive attitude, another important element in fighting cancer.

••• ❖ •••

I have been treating cancer patients since 1984. Patients always have better results when they keep to the treatment plan, follow the diet instructions, maintain a positive attitude toward cancer healing, and exercise regularly.

Part III

Good Health and Longevity

Chapter 7

Chinese Medicine's Secrets of Good Health and Longevity

In China, the way to good health and longevity has always been an intriguing topic. The art of healthful living has evolved through thousands of years into a national tradition. It is quite a surprise to have a strange Chinese person tell someone, "this is healthy and good for you," or "that is not healthy and not good for you." It is very common in Chinese culture to say these things to each other. Health is often discussed, especially in family conversations. Younger people always buy some health-related food or supplement as a gift for their elders when they visit. I remember I used to bring healthy drinks and herbal tonics to my grandparents every time I visited them. Even now, I bring supplements to my mother when I go to China. In our tradition, we never return to visit our families with empty hands, especially when visiting the elderly.

No one can live forever, but people can live longer and happier lives by believing in and practicing traditional Chinese healing arts. Many people think they have good health, but the reality is that they do not.

Trends in Longevity

The secrets of longevity, which sounds somewhat mysterious, have been sought for many centuries. Longevity involves three factors: genetics, lifestyle, and illness. In parts of China, when looking for a life partner, some Chinese still use genetics as a guideline to future health. That means, no matter how good this person is, without good health, the other person might not choose them for their spouse. Regardless of whether it is right or wrong, it certainly points towards the value of health and longevity. Genetic factors play a very important role in longevity. Good lifestyle is also very important; it prolongs the life of a person even without special genes for longevity. Illness, especially a major illness, can reduce the number of years a person will live.

A Japanese geriatric institute spent 10 years studying senior citizens' health. They investigated 422 seniors, all aged around 70 years old, and with decent health. The standards of measure included: individual physical condition, social activity, psychological measure, etc. Eighteen factors were investigated. The outcomes were:

- Overweight or underweight seniors lived shorter lives than those with normal weight.
- Seniors with poor memory lived shorter lives than those with good memory.
- Seniors who do not participate in social activities lived shorter lives than those who participate in all kinds of activities.
- Seniors who were physically strong with good grabbing strength lived longer than weaker people did.*

After researching many different people in different Chinese provinces, Chinese scientists discovered that longevity is related to these factors:

- Healthy mind, open minded, rich in spirit, optimistic with life, kind to people, and have faith in life.
- Healthy diet.
- Fresh air, fresh water.
- Love to work and exercise.
- Appropriate amounts of trace minerals.

What is Good Health?

This is both an easy and a complicated question. Some people think good health means you have good physical stamina, muscle tone, or body figure. I think that good health should include three things: good physical condition, mind and spiritual condition, and social skills and ability. Without any one of these, you cannot say you have good health, because soon you would lose the health you have. Japanese researchers think that good health should have four aspects: good eating, sleeping, eliminating, and speaking.

- Good eating means a healthy person has good appetite, and eats healthy foods.
- Good sleeping means a healthy person has a sufficiently good quality sleep every day.

---

* From *Modern/Ancient Longevity Search*, 2002 Chang Hong Publishing Company, Beijing.

- Good eliminating means a healthy person has good bowel movements and normal urination.
- Good speaking means a healthy person has quick responses and mental alertness.

TCM standards of good health include:
1. Good daily energy level and stamina.
2. Healthy personality.
3. Sleeps well.
4. Good adaptability to natural changes (weather, season); rarely catches cold.
5. Appropriate weight.
6. Appropriate vision and hearing.
7. Strong teeth and bones.
8. Good muscle tone.

Healthy Personality

1. Able to manage stress.
2. Positive attitude.
3. Avoids haggling or disputing about small issues or money.
4. Independent working and living, able to make right decisions.
5. Knows how to love family, relatives, friends, and gets joy from love.
6. Able to receive love or help from friends and family.
7. Good self-control.
8. Goal oriented. Able to give up small things (even things that are beneficial at the present time) in order to reach goals that are usually more valuable. There is a Chinese saying: "Throw sesame away in order to get watermelon."
9. Rest well, not only while sleeping, but also able to rest the mind when doing other leisure or hobby activities.
10. Loves children and provides appropriate education to them. Willing to spend time to find out what children need.
11. Loves to work. Not only enjoys working and staying on the job, but also does not mind doing housework (i.e., is able to find positive aspects of housework).
12. Forgives others for making mistakes.
13. Constantly learning, cultivating spirit and pastimes.

I often joke with people: If you have a good personality, everyone wants to marry you, or everyone wants to be your girlfriend or boyfriend; but actually, it is true that people want to be your friends if you have a good personality.

At first, personality does not seem to have anything to do with health, but it actually does. Individuals have different levels of organ energy and different genes. Some genes contain weaker organ energy than others. For instance, if your mother has weak kidney energy, she might have arthritis in later life, and you are at risk of getting arthritis in your later life, too. If your father has liver energy problem that is related to his depression, you should pay attention to your moods and emotions, because you might have these problems as well. In general, poor personality is related to imbalance of organ energy and imbalance of body chemicals that can cause health problems. Having a poor personality is related to poor childhood education and influence. In this case, vise versa, the poor personality can cause organ energy imbalance. If you know someone who has a poor personality, you know that this person has some sort of imbalance; even while his or her appearance seems fine. Do you know anyone who has a bad personality with good health?

The personality problem can be corrected either with self-study from various sources, including Daoism, or a TCM practitioner can help you to balance your organ energy. Learning is the beginning of correction. Once you open your mind and eyes, you allow the positive energy to come in; the more you learn, the better your outlook will become. When a person stops learning, you know he or she will not change. Keep in mind, change takes time; it does not come within the next day or weeks. It could take a few years to a lifetime. The more open-minded you are, the quicker you will learn.

Tips for Longevity and Balanced Health

After studying centenarians in China, Chinese researchers summed up the following points that have a very close relationship to longevity:

Follow the principles of Yin and Yang

Prevent seasonal diseases by wearing clothes that are appropriate for seasonal changes. During the spring, temperatures change dramatically, so we need to change our clothing dramatically and we are wearing clothing appropriate for the weather. For instance, if the temperature is 50 degrees when you go out but 30 degrees later. If you only plan for the 50-degree weather, you will not have enough clothing on hand when it is colder. The cold would cause an imbalance of your organs; the organ imbalance makes you vulnerable to outside pathogens. You then get a cold or the flu. Therefore, even though it is 50 degrees outside on a nice spring day, you still need to prepare for the worst.

During the spring, the feeling of depression also tends to return. Many people have winter depression, which we call seasonal depression, but spring depression is not uncommon. In Chinese medicine, spring is related to wood, wood is related to liver, which is, and liver energy is related to emotion and mood. Getting out more and enjoying nature will help you to prevent spring depression.

In spring, the air is humid, and pain and aches are more bothersome due to the dampness in the body caused by high humidity; so you should get Chinese herbs or acupuncture treatment. You can also take appropriate medication for symptomatic relief. Because of these seasonal changes, TCM health care offices are generally busier during this time of the year.

Summer is the best time of the year to participate in outdoor activities. Many illnesses improve with regular outdoor activities in the summer. Avoid air conditioning that blows directly on you, especially after you have been sweating, because when the pores of the skin are open, the coldness can go into the body and cause stagnation of blood and energy, resulting in arthritis, muscle aches, and other ailments.

Elderly people should try to avoid ice cold or greasy foods, because many elderly suffer from insufficiency of spleen Yang, which is related to digestion and absorption. They should eat more fruits, vegetables, and other food that are easily digested. Elderly people should pay close attention to their digestive function to avoid many ailments. Walking after dinner can prolong life. There is a Chinese proverb, "By walking 100 steps after dinner, you will live to be 99," thus emphasizing the benefits from walking. The theory is that walking after a meal can help improve digestion.

Some people do not get as much sleep as usual during the summer because nights are shorter. Regarding how much sleep you need, I believe as long as you have enough energy during the day, you are fine, even with fewer hours of sleep. Your body can tell you if you need more sleep.

In the fall, temperatures drop quickly at night and proper attire is important. Relapses from old illnesses occur easily at this time of the year. Good exercise and self-massage is appropriate for maintaining health. In the fall, too, some people have constipation, which is caused from dry air and not drinking enough water. To correct this, I suggest eating more vegetables and fruits. Diarrhea and stomach flu is common as well, most likely from eating raw or contaminated food. Try to eat more cooked food. Do not be surprised if find you hair falling out more than usual. Remember, leaves fall from the trees in the fall, too.

During the winter season, going to bed early and getting up late is fine because nature behaves similarly; days are shorter and nights are longer. Even though most animals are dormant in the winter and you might find your energy level is low, it is better if you continue exercising regularly to preserve energy and vitality. Winter is the season to gain weight, so diet and exercise are extremely important. Many exercises can be done indoors. My school offers exercise classes year round and they are all indoors.

Following the principle of Yin and Yang can help you to adapt to whatever you need to, and make your life much easier and more flexible.

Do exercises best suited to your condition

It does not matter what kind of exercises you do, as long as you exercise, you gain benefits. Choose whatever exercise you like, and do them consistently. Quite a few choice exist such as jogging, walking, going to the gym, playing sports, dancing, aerobics, yoga, Taiji, Qigong, martial arts, etc. I prefer Taiji and Qigong, because they ground my energy, keep me focused, make me feel good, make my body warm, keep my mind clear and calm, and give me a sense of beauty. They also enhance my healing ability and make my healing practice more effective. Yet, no matter how good people say a particular exercise is, you will not do it if you do not like it. You need to find the right exercise regime for you. Most Western exercise promotes blood circulation, whereas most Eastern exercise promotes energy circulation. Both are very important in preserving good health and preventing illness. One type of exercise might be better than another type for some people, but not for everyone. We are all different, so we choose different exercises. Overall, exercise should be a daily activity, a sort of special meal, an energy meal.

Rational diet and moderation in food and drink

The importance of a healthy diet was discussed previously in this book. Diet plays a large part in longevity and a healthy life. There are certain foods that many people are often not using in their diet that have many health benefits. I have seen more and more people willing to try these foods, which is a positive step forward.

Soybean products: The soybean is the king of all beans. Soy products are very healthy foods that provide multiple nutritional benefits. In China, we eat many soybean products. Soybeans are low in cholesterol, high in calcium and phosphates, and many other minerals, including iron. It contains almost all necessary amino acids. Soy protein has almost the same quality as an equal amount of meat. Other lipids in soybean products help to reduce cholesterol and prevent heart disease.

Bean curd, also called tofu, which is made from soybeans, has three times the protein and twice the calcium than milk. Tofu also has five times more phosphate and almost ten times more iron than milk. There is also more magnesium in tofu than milk. One problem for some people is that once they hear that soy is good for their health, they tend to eat too much. Eating too much tofu can cause stomach problems. Remember, anything in extreme will cause an imbalance of body energy.

Sweet potatoes: Scientists have discovered that the sweet potato contains a substance called DHEA (dehydroepiandrosterone), which is similar to adrenaline.

DHEA is a hormone normally produced by the adrenal glands that diminishes as a person ages. DHEA is a precursor to male and female hormones. The scientist did an experiment in which he used a drug to induce cancer in laboratory mice. One group of mice with cancer received an injection of DHEA, and the other group, with the same cancer, did not get the DHEA injections. The mice that were injected with DHEA survived 36 months. The mice without the injection of DHEA survived 24 months.

Green tea: China is the home of tea. Chinese have been drinking tea since the fourth century. By the ninth century, tea drinking was introduced to Japan, and it had spread to Europe by the seventeenth century. Ancient Chinese realized that drinking tea has many health benefits. The ancient Chinese medical book from Qin Dynasty titled: *Shen Nong Ben Cao Jing* recorded this wisdom: "Tea tastes bitter, drink it to improve the mind; dispels laziness, enlivens the body, and brightens the sight." In the Tang Dynasty, culture and education reached a peak and produced many poets. Lu T'ung, a Tang poet wrote this poem about tea drinking:

First cup moistens mouth and throat.

Second cup dispels loneliness and boredom.

Third cup makes the brain quick and lively, capable of writing five thousand volumes.

Fourth cup brings mild perspiration, draining all lifelong grievances through the pores.

Fifth cup refreshes muscles and bones.

Sixth cup brings communion with immortals.

No sooner has one drunk the seventh cup, then a cool breeze lifts one up from below one's arms.

The explanation: First, promotes saliva secretion; second, makes one strong and exhilarated; third, helps digestion and dissolves greasy food; fourth, induces perspiration and cures the common cold; fifth, helps to reducing weight; sixth, invigorates thinking and strengthens memory; seventh, prolongs life. Even though this is just an exaggerative poem and nobody would drink seven cups tea a day, it gives us knowledge about the health benefits in green tea.

Scientists have discovered that tea regulates lipid metabolism, lowers cholesterol, and prevents the accumulation of lipids in vascular walls, therefore maintaining vascular elasticity. The medical school from which I graduated in China (Hunan Medical University) did a study on green tea. They learned that green tea can lead cancer cells to suicide, but the mechanism was unclear. Green tea also helps to combat diabetes; however, it is unclear what the mechanism is that accomplishes this. Tea contains a substance similar to aspirin that can prevent heart disease. This

How to make tasty green tea:
When you make tea, use green tea leaves, not a tea bag. The tea bag is convenient, but nutrients and flavor are lost during processing. Put ½ teaspoon green tea leaves (too much could cause palpitation, insomnia, and constipation) in the teacup. Add 1/3 cup boiled water; let sit for 5 minutes. After the leaves are fully soaked (about 5 minutes), add boiled water to fill the cup. When you drink one cup of the tea, you can add more hot water to make a second cup without adding more tea leaves.

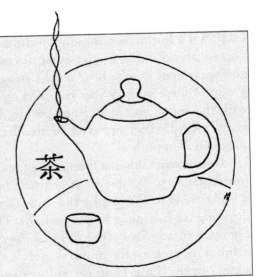

substance might be related to the reduction of blood lipids. The rate of heart disease is lower in China than in the U.S. and even though the average cholesterol level in China is increasing (diet changing), it is still lower than the average in the U.S.

Other Chinese herbal tonics: Chinese herbal tonics are taken primarily for balancing the body's constitution. For instance, if you have too much Yang (energy), which shows itself in symptoms of hot flashes, hypertension, insomnia, and other Yang-type symptoms, you need to take Yin tonics. If you have Yin symptoms, such as being cold all the time, fatigue, diarrhea, and other Yin-type symptoms, you need to take Yang tonics. If you have poor energy, you need to take energy tonics. If you have poor blood, you need to take blood tonics. These conditions should be diagnosed by a qualified TCM practitioner, not by you. Some herbal tonics enhance the immune system, boost energy, nourish the brain and blood, reduce toxins, and others get rid of certain aches and pain. Only a qualified practitioner can prescribe the appropriate tonics for you. Once your body energy is balanced, you do not need the tonics anymore. You do not take tonics for a lifetime. For a healthy person, an herbal tonic would not do much, just as it is not necessary to take vitamins when your body already contains plenty of vitamins because there is simply no need.

For cancer patients, herbal tonics are very beneficial. Selected herbs improve cellular immunity such as *Codonopsis pilosulae* (pilose asiabell root), or Atractylodes (Bai Zu), etc. Other herbs improve the macrophage (a type of white blood cell) capability such as ginseng (Ren Shen), Astragalus (Huang Qi), or *Codonopsis pilosulae* (pilose asiabell root) . Some herbs increase the quantity of antibodies in the body or increase the lymphocyte transformation such as ginseng (Ren Sen), Atractylodes (Bai Zu), Salvia (red sage root), Ligustici (Chuan Xiong, and many other heat clearing detoxifying herbs. Some herbs improve the endurance of antibodies and increase the ability of antibodies to fight disease.

Regular daily schedule

A regular schedule can help maintain better energy flow. Our body has natural timers that recognize our energy pattern. If we disturb the pattern, we lose the natural timer that affects our immune system and other body chemistries, thus causing an imbalance of energy and eventually illness. For instance, if you go to bed at 7 P.M. some days and 2 A.M. on others, you will not only be tired, but you will also soon lose your ability to concentrate or focus. You might even become moody and irritable.

Your mealtimes should be regular, too. A lunch at noon one day and at 3 P.M. another will disturb your stomach energy; the imbalanced stomach energy soon would affect other organ energy, which would eventually cause problems. Unless you choose to, of course, you do not have to have lunch exactly at noon, unless you choose to. You can have your own schedule as long as meals are always around the same time.

The same goes for exercise; it should be regular, too. If you do a heavy physical workout for a period of time, then stop, you will gain weight and increase your chances of getting cardiovascular illness.

Regular times for resting, eating, and exercise are like recharging the battery or refilling the fuel tank of your car. Without these healthy refills of energy, our body will begin to deteriorate sooner. You probably have noticed this for yourself already, but sometimes we lose discipline, which I call an occasional unhealthy habit. If it is really only occasional, then it is acceptable.

Use brain actively and engage in continuous learning

As we get older, our body becomes older. Most people would think the brain gets older, too; however, this is not entirely so. If you do not continue to use the brain, it will get old; but if you do use the brain regularly, constantly recharging this special organ, it could be much younger than your chronological age, even when you are very old. That is why you see some seniors who are very sharp, very bright, and able to perform challenging tasks. Others are very confused and might not even remember what you told them five minutes before.

Many Chinese centenarians are multitalented: they paint, write poems, make wood carvings, practice Chinese calligraphy, play Chinese chess or Go (a game played by many Chinese military). They believe these activities are like Qigong and can improve one's physical and mental health by bringing peace and harmony to the mind. When a calligrapher is using his brush, he naturally concentrates his mind wholly on his subjects and puts aside other thoughts. These activities involve constant learning, too.

Studies have shown that the human brain begins to atrophy after the age of 40. If one uses the brain regularly, however, this process slows down. People who have a family history of Alzheimer's disease need to pay extreme attention to learning. Constant stimulation of the brain could prevent this illness or delay its onset. A number of articles and studies discuss using the brain to prevent senility.

Learning is always rewarding. The more you learn, the smarter you will be, and the better life you will have. No matter how old you are, you can still maintain your sharpness, clearness, cleverness, and "old man's" wisdom. Never lock your mind in a cage, because you will lose a lot of fun and opportunity for fun. Once you say, "I cannot learn," you are begging for your brain to start aging. Learning Taiji and Qigong provides indirect stimulation and prevents aging of the brain. Learning Taiji and Qigong might take a whole lifetime, but it is very beneficial for preventing aging of the brain.

I often tell my children as well as my students, "The day you stop learning is the day you are dead." What I am trying to say is *never stop learning*.

When you retire, you should not completely retire. Doing some volunteer work gives you a sense of being helpful and useful. A patient once asked me, "Why should I do this if I do not get paid?" He did not realize the benefits would come from helping out. Feeling good, in certain circumstances, is much better than money. Certain work involves learning, which is an excellent way to prevent aging of the brain, and being able to help others should be a pleasure.

Conversation is another excellent way to learn. People get together to share their thoughts, ideas, information, and healthy tips such as cooking, sports, sightseeing, and many other enjoyable topics. I talk to people every day in the course of my work, and I feel like I am learning everyday. Get friends together once a while, have a cup of tea or coffee, cake or pastry, have a blast talking about any number of different things.

Keep a peaceful mind

Many physical problems come from a disturbed mind. We deal with stress everyday; this becomes a normal state of life. You will know the normal stress from everyday life because you will not feel too badly; you will just deal with it. When you lose the ability to deal with stress, you will then have a troubled mind, and consequently other problems will come. The peaceful mind enables energy to flow well throughout the body. This smooth energy will help with many things in your life. Studying people over 100 years old in China showed that a majority of them have a peaceful mind, and that they are also open minded, kind, have a positive attitude, are calm, hard working, and do not easily get upset. Many of them, ironically, practice Daoist philosophy but do not even know what Dao is or that that Daoist practice helps a great deal in keeping the mind peaceful.

Tips to keep the mind at peace:
1. Be natural and follow the natural instinct. Do whatever you feel is right for you.

2. Avoid thinking about your physical and emotional problems. The more you think about them, the worse they will get. Do whatever you need to do, such as exercise, make a doctor's appointment, or get help from other professionals.

3. Avoid being obsessed with a financial situation. This creates huge stress. Do whatever you need to do to change the situation.

4. Avoid extreme behaviors (gambling, drugs, alcohol, sweets, overeating, smoking, sleeping, working, and so on). Drinking alcohol occasionally should not cause problems.

5. Add whatever is needed. If you feel sick, take medicine; if you feel hungry, eat food or a snack; if you need supplements, go get them; and if you are tired, rest.

6. Avoid conflicts with people, law, property, etc. Conflict causes major stress in life and disturbs the mind.

7. Avoid comparing. It does not matter who is better, who is richer, who has the better house or car, or who is smarter. We all have our own special roles, our own special enjoyment for life.

Proper self-care and nourishment: Many people in China do self-massage to maintain good health. Self-massage improves the immune system, circulation, metabolism, and digestive system. It also delays aging. It is like an energy nutrition that nourishes the body. It also helps to relieve discomfort, such as headaches, insomnia, neck problems, stomach pain, diabetes, and so forth.

As previously discussed, proper self-care includes exercise, self-massage, herbal tonics or appropriate supplements, appropriate diet and nutrition.

Fresh air and a beautiful environment

We need to do more work or activities outdoors; breathing fresh air gives us more oxygen. Every form of life needs oxygen. In the wintertime, when we are not able to do many outdoor activities, we feel down and depressed. Lack of sunlight is one reason for seasonal depression, and lack of oxygen is another reason. Sufficient oxygen is very important for maintaining good health and preventing aging. In China, many centenarians live in rural areas with abundant fresh air and natural beautiful, environments. The centenarians who live in the city like to plant flowers on the balcony or go to parks in the morning to exercise. Luckily, there are many beautiful parks in big/midsized cities, in every state and country.

Flowers are considered by some people as a natural tranquilizer. They soothe the body and mind and bring positive energy to the body. You just feel good when you look at flowers. Planting flowers can relieve stress and is very easy to do. I dislike winter, partly because the flowers in my garden are all dead during the winter. I take many pictures in the summertime, so that I can still enjoy my flowers during the winter months.

Family harmony

I know this is easier said than done but maintaining family harmony requires much constant work, but it is very beneficial for our health. Understanding a person is like understanding nature. Once you understand, your tolerance level will be higher, you will get along better, and you will not say hurtful things or be defensive when someone else says the wrong things. A harmonious family creates a warm nest in which you can relax, rejuvenate, take shelter from the storm, have fun, get rid of stress, cuddle, and enjoy a more peaceful life.

Many health problems come from dysfunctional family dynamics. When you have family disharmony, you might try to find outside help to bring balance to the situation.

Little problems can be solved on a daily or weekly basis. With appropriate methods, the big issues will become small issues, and the small issues will not be issues at all. You can then have a good night's sleep. Good family values are very important and are necessary to the familial teamwork required to win life's battles. Everyone in the family is responsible for building strong family relationships.

> A patient once told me that her mother died from cancer within one year after diagnosis. The doctor diagnosed her constant rectal bleeding problem as hemorrhoids. When the bleeding finally caught the doctor's attention, it was too late. She had end-stage colon cancer. Early diagnosis is extremely important, especially for treating cancer.
>
> Another patient had shoulder pain, and she assumed it would get better. After many years, scar tissue built up and she could not move the arm, then she had to have surgery.

Avoid overexertion

Any kind of overexertion is not healthy. Overwork depletes your overall energy level; too much sex can be harmful to your kidney energy; overeating can harm your stomach energy; excessive drinking can harm liver energy; being overly anxious can harm heart energy, and so on. Longevity comes from a balanced and healthy lifestyle. Some people think that more the better, whereas I think the less the better, because there would be less about which to worry (although I could be wrong). In modern day life, the less the better might not be practical. If you do not care about how long you live, you choose to do whatever you want; even if what you do is harmful to your health, but at least you enjoy it at the moment. During the time of leading an unhealthy life, tell people who worry and care about you that it was my choice and not to worry Otherwise, the worry can harm their health, which means your choice might affect the lives of others.

Seek medical help at an early stage

In many cases, people suffer from major health problems resulting from missed early diagnosis and treatment.

Acute illnesses are easy to treat, and take less time to treat; chronic illness, on the other hand, take much more time to treat and are more difficult to treat. Chronic problems are also expensive to treat and decrease the overall lifespan.

Go to a doctor you like, it does not matter whether it is Western or Eastern medicine. Go to Western medicine first, because it is more accessible, but if the Western medicine does not help, you should try Chinese medicine. It is safe, effective, and a true healing methodology.

Building a Bridge to a Wonderful Life

We live in a fast-paced society and deal with stress almost every day. If we choose the way of living wisely, our life will not only last longer but also be happier. When you look back, life is very short. We cannot afford to lose even one day. We need to make everyday life valuable and cherished. We need to learn to build a bridge to a good life. The day when you reach the end of your life, you will be still satisfied with what you have done, you will be proud of yourself for being able to live to the end with fullness of life.

Have a great life!

Appendixes

Commonly Used Patent Herbs and Herbal Tonics

There is a large population of Asians who use herbal tonics regularly when they reach a certain age. These are patent herb preparations, regulated by the Chinese government for many years, which are considered effective with no side effects. Some people use herbs only when they have minor ailments, which I consider is better than taking them for a long time. There are some commonly used herb tonics in certain areas in the United States in TCM herbal pharmacies or even Chinese markets. Many TCM practitioners give these herbs to patients. Once you become familiar with these herbs, when your TCM practitioner prescribes these herbs, you would feel more comfortable than taking something you do not know.

Patented Herbs and Herbal Tonics

Problem	Recommended Herb Tonics
Flu and Colds	Yin Qiao Jie Du Pian
	Ban Lan Gen
	Gan Mao Ching
	Gan Mao Ling
	Chuan Xin Lian
Sinus	Bi Yan Pian
	Bi Ming Gan Wan
Chronic Lung Problems	Li Fei Pian
	Ma Xin Zi Ke Pian
Indigestion and Poor Appetite	Bao He Wan
	Jian Pi Wan
Depression	Xiao Yao WanBai Zi Yang Xin Wan
	Shu Gan Wan
Hot Flashes	Zi Bai Di Huang Wan
Menopause	Ji Ju Di Huang Wan
	Liu Wei Di Huang Wan

Recipes for Healthy Eating, Asian Style

Chinese Meat Sauce (chicken or beef)

Serves 6

If you are a meat eater, you should eat meat in small portions and cook meat in different ways. Cooking meat in this sauce can reduce fat, balance the organs, and add additional flavor. It is one of the most delicious ways to prepare meats.

Ingredients:
2 pounds meat
1 dried orange peel
3 star anise
1 cinnamon bark (stick)
5 green onions (white head)
1 teaspoon fennel
3 dried red hot peppers
¼ teaspoon black pepper
1 teaspoon chopped ginger
1 whole garlic
½ teaspoon salt

Wash the meat, put meat in a pot with water, add all of the above ingredients, and bring to a boil. Once boiling, reduce heat to low and let simmer for 50 minutes to one hour. Remove the meat, cut it to desired size, and discard the soup. This way you do not consume the chemicals in the meat. The various spices not only make the meat more flavorful, but also balance the organs.

After cooking the meat, you can either cut and eat it, or cut it in to small pieces and marinate with soy sauce, vinegar, sesame oil, hot pepper sauce, and garlic. You can also cut the meat and mix with salad.

Vegetarian Sushi Wrap
Serves 1

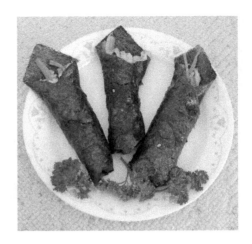

Ingredients:
sushi wrap
cooked rice with a little salt, a little
    vinegar, and sugar
chopped lettuce
chopped scallion
1 sliced avocado
dash of catsup or soy sauce
salt and pepper, to taste

Lay sushi wrap on table, put rice on the wrap first, and then all ingredients in the center of the wrap. Roll the wrap and then eat with your fingers. If you eat meat, you can use sliced ham to substitute for rice and add a little mayonnaise.

Chinese Tofu (Bean Curd) Soup
Serves 4 to 5

Ingredients:
3 Chinese dried mushrooms
1 ounce dried lily flower (optional)
6 fresh mushrooms
2 ounces baby shrimp (optional) or dried shrimp
1 firm tofu
1 tablespoon starch
$1/8$ teaspoon salt
$1/8$ teaspoon pepper
1 teaspoon soy sauce
2 bouillon cubes
1 scallion, chopped
2 cups water

Soak the dried mushrooms for 10 minutes, and then wash them. Cut the mushrooms into small pieces. Place both types of mushrooms, bouillon cubes, shrimp, salt, soy sauce, and tofu in the water, and bring to a boil. Mix starch with ½ cup water, put the mix into the soup to thicken it. Put soup into a large bowl and add scallion and pepper. Mix and serve.

Vegetable Stir-Fry

Serves 3 to 4

Ingredients:
2 zucchini
2 carrots
1 green pepper
3 garlic cloves
½ teaspoon salt
1 teaspoon soy sauce (optional)
2 tablespoon vegetable or olive oil

Cut all vegetables into 2 inch strings. Put two tablespoons of vegetable or olive oil in a wok or frying pan; put the chopped garlic into wok, put all vegetables in the wok and stir-fry for 5 minutes. If the stir-fry is too dry, add a little water. Add salt. Soy sauce is optional. You can try using the soy sauce one time, and not using it another time. You can also use less salt, if you prefer.

Vegetarian Pocket

Serves 1

Ingredients:
1 pita bread
½ onion
6 mushrooms
½ green pepper
½ cup lettuce
1 teaspoon teriyaki sauce
1 tablespoon olive oil
sea salt and pepper, to taste

Cut onion, green pepper, and lettuce into thin strings. Slice the mushrooms. Cook onion, pepper, and mushrooms in olive oil, and add salt and pepper or a little teriyaki sauce, or both. Cut lettuce into thin strings but not cooked. Put lettuce and cooked vegetables inside the pita bread. If you like hot spicy foods, add some hot sauce to the pocket.

Chinese Noodles with Spice, Meat, and Vegetables

Serves 4

Ingredients:
1 pound wide noodles
1 bunch scallions
½ pound beef or chicken
1 teaspoon chopped ginger
¼ cabbage
¼ pound bean sprouts
¼ cup chopped cilantro (Chinese parsley)
1 teaspoon sesame oil
3 tablespoons soy sauce
1/8 teaspoon pepper
3 tablespoons olive or vegetable oil
½ teaspoon salt
hot sauce for those who like spicy foods

Cook the noodles until soft. Drain the noodles and put aside after cooking. Meanwhile, prepare the vegetable mix.

Chop the cabbage thin, wash and chop the scallion to a quarter inch, and separate white and green parts. Chop the cilantro to ½ inch pieces. Cut meat to 1½ to 2 inch strings and mix with 1 tablespoon soy sauce. Wash the bean sprouts and drain.

Put 3 tablespoons olive oil or vegetable oil in wok or frying pan on stove over high heat. Put chopped ginger and white parts of the scallion in the wok, then put chopped meat into wok and stir-fry until meat is fully cooked. Add cabbage to the wok, add salt and stir-fry with other ingredients. Put this mix into a big bowl, add cooked noodles, green parts of the scallion, bean sprouts, chopped cilantro, 1 teaspoon sesame oil, 2 teaspoons soy sauce, and pepper. Add hot sauce if you like spicy foods.

Carrots and Daikon String Mix (Salad)

Serves 4 to 6

Ingredients:
1 pound daikon (Chinese radish)
½ pound carrots
½ bunch scallions
½ teaspoon salt
2 tablespoons vinegar
1 tablespoon sugar
1 teaspoon sesame oil

Cut daikon, carrots, and scallions to thin strings and put in a bowl. Add salt, mix the vegetables, and then leave for 10 minutes. Discard the liquid; add vinegar, sugar, and sesame oil; mix and let set for 5 minutes. Enjoy the delicious and nutritious salad.

Eggplant Shi-Chuan Style

Serves 4 to 6

Ingredients:
4 Oriental eggplants or two regular eggplants
½ teaspoon chopped ginger
1 teaspoon chopped garlic
1 tablespoon hot bean paste
2 tablespoons soy sauce
1 tablespoon vinegar
1 teaspoon sugar
1 teaspoon salt
½ teaspoon sesame oil
6 tablespoons oil
1 tablespoon chopped green onion

Choose firm, purple eggplants, remove the stalk, and cut into thumb-sized pieces. Heat the oil in a frying pan until very hot. Put eggplant in the pan, turn heat to low, stir-fry until the eggplant is soft (about 3 minutes). Then squeeze out the excess oil. Remove eggplant from pan and set aside. Into the frying pan, add chopped garlic, ginger, and hot bean paste, stir a few seconds, and add soy sauce, sugar, and salt. Add eggplant and cook until the sauce is almost gone. Add vinegar and sesame oil, and stir until heated through. Sprinkle with chopped green onion. Mix and serve.

Spareribs and Bean Sprout Soup

Serves 8

Ingredients:
½ pounds spareribs
9 cups water
2 pieces of ginger
¼ pound bean sprouts
1 small tomato
1 teaspoon salt
1 piece scallion, chopped

Put spareribs, water, ginger, small tomato, and salt together and boil for 40 minutes. Add bean sprouts and boil for 15 more minutes. Sprinkle scallion afterwards.

Sweet and Sour Spareribs

Serves 6

Ingredients:
1¼ pounds spareribs
3 green onions
4 tablespoons soy sauce
4 tablespoons sugar
3 tablespoons vinegar
5 tablespoons cold water
2 tablespoons cornstarch
1 tablespoon cooking wine
1 tablespoon sesame oil
3 tablespoons oil

Cut the spareribs into 1 inch square pieces, then marinate with wine and soy sauce for 30 minutes. Deep-fry the spareribs for about 5 minutes, until spareribs turn brown. Remove spareribs and drain oil from frying pan. Add sugar, vinegar, water, and cornstarch, sesame oil, and shredded green onion to the bowl used for marinating spareribs. This is the seasoning sauce. Heat one tablespoon oil in frying pan, pour in the seasoning sauce, boil and stir until thickened and heated thoroughly; add spareribs and stir well before serving.

Shi-Chuan Cucumber

Serves 2 to 3

Ingredients:
1¼ pounds cucumbers (about 7 pieces)
15 slices garlic
1 teaspoon Shi-Chuan pepper (crushed)
1 teaspoon hot bean paste
1 teaspoon hot oil
1 teaspoon salt
2 teaspoons sugar
1 teaspoon vinegar
2 teaspoons sesame oil

Cut off and discard both tips of cucumbers, then cut into diagonal or triangular shapes. Put them and ½ teaspoon salt in a bowl, soak for 30 minutes. Wash the cucumber with cold water and let dry. Put it back in bowl. Add garlic slices, Shi-Chuan pepper, hot bean paste, hot oil, sugar, vinegar, and sesame oil. Mix and soak about 30 minutes.

Vegetarian Soup

Serves 4 to 6

Ingredients:
1 cup adzuki beans, washed and soaked for 6 to 8 hours, or overnight (save
    soaking water)
2 inch square pieces kelp
1 cup onions, diced
1 cup winter squash (buttercup, red kori, butternut, etc.)
2 carrots, sliced
½ cup corn kernels
5 cups water
½ teaspoon sea salt
2 scallions, chopped for garnish

Soak the kelp for 30 minutes and then wash it. Place beans (including soaking water), water, and kelp into a pot. Cover and bring to a boil over high heat. Reduce heat to medium low and simmer for 1½ hours.

Add vegetables and salt. Continue cooking for another 30 minutes.

Remove from heat. Sprinkle scallions over top and serve.

Quick Sautéed Greens

Serves 4 to 6

Ingredients:
4 cups greens (kale, collards, etc.)
1 tablespoon olive oil
3 pieces garlic
½ teaspoon sea salt
½ teaspoon sesame oil
hot pepper (optional)

Wash greens well, drain, and cut into bite-sized pieces, or in one inch lengths.
Place oil in pan and heat on medium high. Add minced garlic and sauté; then add other greens and sauté until half cooked, about 4 minutes.

Other Oriental Vegetarian Recipes

The recipes below are from Cid Shane, an American-born of Japanese descent who has a passion for health and a vegetarian diet for both humans and animals. In the past, she offered a cooking class in my school and had a wonderful reputation for her personality and cooking professionalism. I took her cooking class and learned many wonderful vegetarian dishes, such as California roll (a type of sushi), Vietnamese spring roll, rice salad, miso soup, etc. Some of them I still use regularly because they are easy to make, tasty, low in calories, and add a variety of nutrition to my diet. With her passion for healthy eating and cooking, she left quite an impression with my students.

Japanese Sushi

Ingredients for California Rolls:
nori (seaweed sheets), "toasted"
Japanese short-grained white rice
1 avocado, peeled, pitted, and cut into strips
1 cucumber, scrubbed, and cut into 1/16 to 1/8 inch strips
1 carrot, scrubbed, and cut into 1/16 to 1/8 inch strips (slightly cooked)

Ingredients for Nori Maki
nori (toasted seaweed sheets)
short-grained white rice
seasoned rice vinegar, 1 tablespoon per 4 cups rice
takewon (pickled daikon) cut into 1/8 inch strips

Ingredients for Vegi Rolls:
nori (toasted seaweed sheets)
short-grained brown rice
asparagus, (ideally) steamed, but can used canned
1 carrot and 1 zucchini cut into 1/16 to 1/8 inch strips
slightly toasted sesame seeds, optional

Cook the rice. Use warm rice, not hot, or nori will shrivel. Sprinkle vinegar over rice; fluff with fork.

Place nori, rough side up and shiny side down, on mat, lining up the bottom edge of the nori with the mat. With dampened fingers, spread a thin layer of rice over entire surface of nori. (I use approximately 1 cup of rice per roll.) Place your chosen fillings at the bottom of the sheet of nori approximately 1/2" to 1" from the edge. Place your thumbs under edge of mat closest to you, with your index fingers resting lightly on your "filling." Roll nori over your "filling"; lift top edge of mat so it does not roll into the nori, and continue to roll. Shape nori inside mat; roll may be either round or square.

To serve, place roll, seam side down, on a cutting board. Using a damp knife (like a serrated knife), to slice the roll into 8 to 10 pieces.

Stir-fried Vegetables and Tempeh with Spicy Peanut Sauce
Serves 4 to 6

Sauce:
¼ cup garlic cloves, peeled
¼ cup coarsely chopped, peeled fresh ginger
1 cup smooth peanut butter
½ cup peanut oil
½ cup orange juice
½ cup tamari or soy sauce
⅓ cup honey
¼ cup vinegar
1 tablespoon sesame oil
1 teaspoon chili powder
⅛ to ¼ teaspoon cayenne

To prepare the sauce, process the garlic and ginger in a food processor until finely chopped. Add the peanut butter, peanut oil, orange juice, tamari, honey, vinegar, sesame oil, chili powder, and cayenne, and process until smooth. Put sauce in a saucepan to heat.

To complete the dish:
6 tablespoons canola oil
1 pound tempeh, cut into small triangles
4 tablespoons tamari or soy sauce
24 ounces dry curly pasta
8 cups chopped broccoli (florets sliced)
4 medium carrots, peeled and cut into matchstick shape (2 cups)
4 cups sliced bok choy (8 stalks)
2 large red peppers, seeded and thinly sliced (2 cup)
4 cups chopped zucchini (2 large zucchini)
Put a large pot of water on to boil.

Heat 4 tablespoons of the canola oil in a skillet over medium heat. Sauté the tempeh until lightly browned on all sides, about 10 minutes. Pour the tamari and stir quickly to distribute it. Transfer the tempeh to a large serving bowl.

Heat the peanut sauce over very low heat, stirring occasionally. Cook the pasta in the boiling water until al dente, 8 to 10 minutes.

Meanwhile, heat the remaining 2 tablespoons canola oil in the skillet over medium heat. Sauté the broccoli and carrots for 2 to 3 minutes. Add the bok choy, red pepper, and zucchini, and cook until just tender, 3 to 4 minutes. Add the tempeh and cook just until warmed through, 1 to 2 minutes more. Transfer to a serving bowl.

Drain the pasta, and toss it with the tempeh and vegetables. Add all but a few tablespoons of the hot peanut sauce and toss again. Pour on the reserved sauce and serve.

Chinese Vegetable Stir-Fry (improvisational)

A wonderful stir-fry that is quick, easy, and very flexible. The vegetables can be varied according to your taste.

Serves 4 to 6

Ingredients:

4 teaspoons peanut oil
1 large onion, cut in half, then thinly sliced
½ cup red bell pepper strips
1 cup vegetable broth
1 cup fresh or frozen broccoli florets
1 cup baby carrots or carrots sliced into 1/8 inch slices
1 cup sugar snap peas
5 to 6 mushrooms, thickly sliced
1 small can water chestnuts (sliced)
4 scallions (white and light green parts), slivered
4 tablespoons grated fresh ginger
2 teaspoons red pepper flakes, or to taste
5 tablespoons hoisin sauce
2 pounds firm or baked tofu, well drained and cut into strips

In a wok or large, heavy skillet, heat oil over medium-high heat.

Add onion and bell pepper, and stir-fry 1 minute. Add broth and bring to a boil. Add broccoli, carrots, sugar snap peas, mushrooms, water chestnuts, and scallions and stir-fry 2 minutes. Add ginger, red pepper flakes; cover and cook until vegetables are crisp-tender, about 2 minutes.

Meanwhile, in a small bowl, mix hoisin sauce and 2½ tablespoons water until well blended. Add to stir-fry and mix gently, then add tofu strips and toss gently. Cook, stirring occasionally, just until heated through. Serve right away.

Spicy Rice and Vegetable Salad

Serves 8

Sesame-Chili Dressing:
½ cup rice wine vinegar
½ cup soy sauce (preferably tamari)
¼ cup Asian-style sesame oil
¼ cup hot chili oil, or to taste
¼ cup freshly squeezed lime juice

In a jar with a cover, combine ingredients. Cover and shake to blend well.

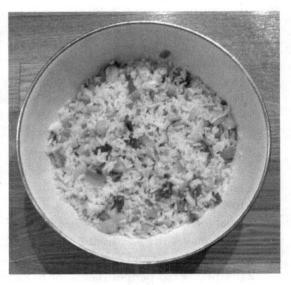

Spicy Rice and Vegetable Salad:
2 cups long-grain white rice
6 green onions, sliced
2 carrots, peeled and diced
1 sweet red pepper, diced
1 to 2 teaspoons minced fresh chili pepper, or to taste
½ cup chopped fresh mint
¼ cup chopped fresh cilantro
⅓ cup chopped unsalted peanuts
2 cups fresh bean sprouts

Garnish with cilantro sprigs. Serve at room temperature.

Cook 2 cups rice in 3 cups water. Fluff with a fork, transfer to a large mixing bowl, and cool slightly. Gently toss the warm rice with about one-third of the dressing. Fluff frequently until the rice cools completely.

Add green onions, carrots, sweet pepper, chili pepper, mint, and cilantro, and toss with the remaining dressing. Place in a serving dish and sprinkle with peanuts, surround with bean sprouts, and garnish with cilantro sprigs.

Miso Soup Variations:

Miso soup never needs to be humdrum. In addition to the classic elements and those called for in the preceding recipes, many ingredients are used to vary the daily bowl. When mixing and matching ingredients, consider visual appeal.

Main Ingredients:

adzuki beans, cooked

cabbage, finely shredded

carrot, thinly sliced and parboiled

daikon, cut into rounds, half moons, or julienne strips, and parboiled

sweet potato, peeled, thinly sliced and parboiled

tofu, grilled

spinach leaves (baby leaves are best)

miso paste

Red Miso Soup

In the classic, most common version of miso soup, shitake mushrooms provide a fancy touch to the everyday red miso and tofu.

Serves 4

Ingredients:

3½ cups vegetable dashi (broth)

3 to 4 tablespoons red miso

½ inch thick slice (about 4 ounces) soft tofu, cut into ½ inch cubes

1 scallion, trimmed and cut into 2 inch long slivers

2 fresh shitake or equal amount of other fresh mushrooms, rinsed, stemmed, and cut into ¼ inch slices

Divide the tofu and scallions among 4 bowls and set aside.

Put the dashi in a medium pot and bring to a boil. Place the miso in a small bowl; before the dashi boils, add ½ cup of the warm dashi, and whisk to smooth.

Add the mushrooms to the dashi and simmer until soft and heated through, about 1 minute. Stir in the miso mixture, taking care not to let the liquid boil again. Ladle the broth and mushrooms into the bowls, and serve right away.

Soup should be warm but not hot. Do not boil as boiling destroys the beneficial enzymes in the miso.

White Miso Soup

White miso, sometimes called temple miso, is sweeter than red and more expensive. It is the kind preferred in Buddhist and Kaiseki (Zen Buddhist) cooking, and for company.

Serves 4

Ingredients:

4 ounces soft tofu, cut into ½ inch cubes or 8 thin slices tofu puffs (*aburage*)

3½ cups vegetable dashi (broth)

1 small or ½ large leek, white part only, trimmed and sliced into very thin rounds, well rinsed

5 to 6 tablespoons white miso

12 strands (1½ inches long) of lemon zest

If using aburage, place the tofu puffs slices in a colander and pour boiling water over them. Set aside.

Put the dashi in a medium pot and bring to a boil.

Place the miso in a small bowl; before the dashi boils, add ½ cup of the warm dashi and whisk to smooth. Set aside.

Add the aburage (if using) or the soft tofu slices and leeks to the main pot of dashi and simmer very gently for 2 minutes until wilted. Stir in the miso, taking care not to let the liquid boil again.

Ladle into soup bowls, dividing the ingredients equally. Garnish with the lemon zest and serve right away.

Non-Traditional Miso Soup

Serves 6 to 8 as a meal

Ingredients:

3 cups cauliflower, sliced (1 small head)
1 cups carrots, sliced (2 carrots)
1½ cups zucchini, quartered and sliced
1 cup green onions, chopped
7 to 8 mushrooms, sliced
1 large bunch spinach, chopped
½ to ¾ block extra firm tofu, cut into ½ inch cubes
1 handful of bean sprouts
5 tablespoons red miso
3 cups frozen peas

Bring 8 cups water to a rapid boil. Add cauliflower and carrots and cook on high for 2½ to 3 minutes.

Add zucchini, green onions, and mushroom and cook on high for 1½ minutes. Remove from heat and add chopped spinach, bok choy or watercress.

Add cubed tofu and bean sprouts; put the lid on the pot, and let it sit approximately 2 minutes.

Add 3 cups peas (frozen) and after soup has cooled from adding the frozen peas, stir in 5 tablespoons red miso to taste. Stir until miso has dissolved.

Soup should be warm but not hot. Do not boil as boiling destroys the beneficial enzymes in the miso.

Easy Vegetables in Curry Sauce

Serves 4 to 6

Ingredients:
2 medium onions cut into 1 inch pieces (approximately 1 cup)
2½ cups organic vegetable broth
4 potatoes cut in ½ inch pieces (approximately 4)
3 carrots sliced in ¼ inch slices (approximately 2 to 3 cups)
8 ounces peas – (½ bag)
14.5 ounce extra firm tofu cut into ½ inch cubes
5 to 7 tablespoons mild curry paste

Sauté onions in a small amount of vegetable or olive oil in a non-stick pan. Add vegetable broth, potatoes, carrots, and peas. and cook until vegetables are tender. Add mild curry paste and stir until dissolved. Add tofu cubes and cook until heated through. Serve vegetables in curry sauce over a bowl of steamed rice.

Other vegetable that lend themselves to curry:
cauliflower
sugar peas
zucchini
baby corn

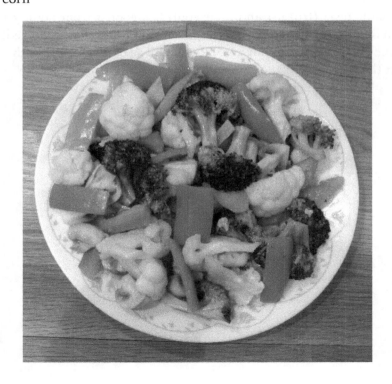

Basic Japanese Vegetable Curry - Donburi

Serves 3

Ingredients:
1 onion, diced (approximately 1 cup)
2 tablespoons vegetable oil
1 potato cut in ½ inch pieces (approximately 1 cup)
1 carrot sliced in ¼ inch slices (approximately 1 cup)
2 cups vegetable stock or water
1 tablespoon shoyu (Japanese soy sauce)
1 teaspoon sugar
1 teaspoon finely minced ginger
1 to 3 tablespoons Japanese curry powder (depending or level of "spicy")
2 tablespoons cornstarch
1 to 2 scallions, chopped (for garnish)
8 ounce peas (optional)
14½ ounce extra firm tofu cut into ½ inch cubes (optional)

Brown onions in oil and sauté until tender. Add the stock, shoyu, sugar, ginger, carrots, and potatoes. Cook until vegetables are tender.

Make a paste of the curry powder with a little water (this will avoid lumps of curry powder in the pot, which are very difficult to break up) and add, stirring briskly to avoid lumps. Add tofu if desired and heat through.

When thickened, serve over hot noodles or steamed white Japanese short-grained rice in a bowl (donburi). Garnish with scallions.

Asian Noodle Salad

Serves 4 to 6

Asian-style vinaigrette:
$1/3$ cup rice wine vinegar
1 teaspoon sugar (optional)
$1/2$ teaspoon salt
$1/2$ teaspoon ground pepper
$1/4$ cup soy sauce (preferably tamari)
1 tablespoon minced fresh ginger root
1 teaspoon minced or pressed garlic
$1/2$ cup oil, equal parts Asian-style sesame oil, high quality vegetable oil and hot chili oil (less chili oil, less heat!)

In a jar with a cover, combine ingredients. Cover and shake to blend well. Use immediately or let stand at room temperature for as long as overnight. Makes a little less than 1 cup.

Asian Noodle Salad:
4 quarts water
1 tablespoon salt (approximately)
1 pound Asian wheat noodles or dried thin Italian spaghetti
8 ounces snow peas, cut on the diagonal into rectangles
1 cup green onions, finely chopped
1 cup unsalted dry-roasted peanuts, coarsely chopped
$1/2$ cup fresh cilantro, chopped

Bring water to a rapid boil and add salt. Add the dried Asian wheat noodles (I use Japanese soba noodles) and cook, stirring frequently until barely tender and still quite firm to the bite, 5 to 8 minutes for dried noodles. Drain, rinse quickly under cold running water, and drain again. Transfer the noodles to a large bowl, add about half of the vinaigrette, and toss well. Cool to room temperature.

Bring to a boil a large saucepan of water, add the snow peas and cook until tender-crisp, about 1 minute. Drain, and then plunge into ice water to halt cooking and preserve color. Drain well.

Add the snow peas, green onion, peanuts, cilantro, and the remaining vinaigrette to the noodles and toss gently but firmly. Serve at room temperature.

Vegetables in Spicy Curry Sauce—Donburi

Chunks of vegetable in a spicy curry sauce sitting on a bed of fluffy steamed rice.
Serves 8

Ingredients:
Boil in 2½ cups water:
2 onions cut into 1 inch pieces (approximately 2 cups)
4 potatoes cut in ½ inch pieces (approximately 4 cups)
2 carrots sliced in ¼ inch slices (approximately 2 to 3 cups)
8 ounce peas (½ bag)

Cid Shane's spicy curry sauce:
3 teaspoon curry powder
1 teaspoon coriander
1 teaspoon Garam masala
½ teaspoon turmeric
½ teaspoon cumin
2 teaspoon arrowroot powder
1 to 2 tablespoons tamari or Japanese soy sauce
¼ cup organic vegetable broth

First mix all dry spices and arrowroot powder (or cornstarch) in a bowl, and add a small amount of the liquid ingredients to make a paste to avoid lumps of curry powder in the pot, which are very difficult to break up. Add liquid ingredients, stirring briskly to avoid lumps. Add sauce to cooked vegetables and adjust thickness with arrowroot power.

Serve the vegetables in a spicy curry sauce over a bowl (donburi) of steamed rice. Traditionally, this is served over Japanese short-grained white rice but can be served over a short-grained brown rice.

Thai Tofu Stew

Thai improvisational, a healthy, yummy stew that can stand on its own or can be served with cooked rice or rice noodles.

Serves 3 to 4

Ingredients:

14 ounce can light coconut milk
1 cup water or vegetable broth
1 pound extra firm tofu, drained and diced
2 tablespoons fresh ginger, minced
6 cloves garlic, minced
6 scallions, chopped
¼ teaspoon red pepper flakes
5 ounce shitake mushrooms, stemmed and diced (2 cups)
2 medium carrots, thinly sliced (1 cup)
1 cup peeled and diced butternut squash
4 cups slivered bok choy
½ cup chopped fresh cilantro

In a large saucepan, combine coconut milk, water or broth, tofu, half the ginger, half the garlic, half the scallions, and red pepper flakes. Bring to a boil, reduce heat to low, and simmer 20 minutes. Turn off the heat.

Transfer 1½ cups of the coconut milk mixture to a large pot. Add mushrooms, carrots, squash, remaining ginger, garlic, and scallions. Cover and simmer over medium heat until vegetables are just tender, about 5 minutes.

Add bok choy to pot and stir just until it begins to wilt, about 45 to 50 seconds. Add cilantro.

Pour remaining coconut mixture over cooked vegetables and stir gently to combine and distribute tofu evenly. Serve hot. Can be served with cooked rice noodles or steamed rice.

Vietnamese Spring Rolls

Vietnamese "salad" rolled in rice paper and served with a peanut dipping sauce.
Serves 6 to 8

Ingredients:

½ to 1 cup carrots
½ to 1 cup zucchini

Cut both into same size matchsticks and steam until still slightly crunchy.
1 cup bean sprouts
½ to 1 cup mint leaves (pick off and use only leaves)
1½ cup lettuce-shredded
Thin rice vermicelli cooked per package instructions
8 to 10 rounds of Vietnamese rice paper (banh trang)

Optional ingredients:
½ to 1 fresh cilantro, chopped
4 scallions, cut into 3 inch pieces, then shredded lengthwise
¼ cup red bell pepper, seeded and finely shredded
½ cup cucumber, seeded, unpeeled, and cut into matchsticks
¾ cup tofu, cut into long cubes (use raw, or fried approximately 2 minutes in a non-stick pan)

Simple peanut sauce (approximately 1 cup):
1 tablespoon vegetable oil (or use a non-stick pan and skip the oil)
½ cup vegetable broth (or water)
½ teaspoon sugar
2 tablespoons peanut butter
¼ cup hoisin sauce
1 or 2 scallions or green onions, thinly sliced

If using oil, heat in a small saucepan. When the oil is hot, add chopped scallions, fry for a couple of minutes. Add the broth, sugar, and peanut butter. Bring to a boil. Reduce the heat and simmer for 3 minutes. Serve warm or at room temperature.

If you are preparing the spring rolls for you or your family and friends, prepare all the ingredients you choose to use as directed and arrange in groups on a board so you can make your spring rolls assembly-style. If you are preparing spring rolls for a party, and wish to have guests make their own spring rolls, place your chosen ingredients in individual bowls.

Have a basin of warm water ready to moisten the rice papers. Immerse each sheet of rice paper into the warm water, leaving immersed long enough to soften and turn white, about 40 seconds, and then carefully lift out and spread on a damp cloth.

Lay lettuce over the bottom third of the rice paper. On the lettuce, place a couple strands of rice noodles, bean sprouts, and several mint leaves. Roll up the rice paper halfway into a cylinder. Fold both ends of the paper over the filling. Place the rolls on a plate and cover with a damp towel so that they will stay moist while you fill the remaining wrappers. Pour the peanut sauce into small individual bowls and sprinkle with the ground peanuts. Dip the rolls in the sauce as you eat.

Marvelous Miso Recipes

Green Beans in Sesame/Miso:
Serves 4

Ingredients:
3 cups fresh green beans, cut on diagonal into 1½ inch lengths
pinch of sea salt
3 tablespoons sesame seeds
1 teaspoon light sesame oil
1 teaspoon lemon juice
2 tablespoons barley, red, or brown rice miso
1 tablespoon mirin (optional)
1 tablespoon brown rice syrup

Place green beans and salt in boiling water and cook, uncovered, until just tender. Drain and cool. Toast sesame seeds in a dry skillet, stirring constantly over medium heat for about 2 minutes, until they are fragrant or begin to pop. Grind seeds in a suribachi or mortar and pestle, add oil and mix, and then add miso and mix. Stir in mirin, lemon juice, and rice syrup, and then toss beans in the liquid until evenly coated.

Shitake-Udon Broth:
Makes approximately 2 servings
2 cups water
1 bundle udon noodles
3 to 4 shiitake mushrooms
2 inch piece wakame
8 to 10 half-inch cubes fresh tofu
1 to 2 teaspoons mellow barley miso or traditional red miso
½ to 1 teaspoon tamari or soy sauce
½ to 1 teaspoon toasted sesame oil

Soak shitakes ½ to 1 hour in 2 cups water. Remove, discard stems, and slice. Return to soaking water, add wakame and tofu pieces, and bring to a full boil. Add udon noodles and cook, uncovered, for 5 to 6 minutes, or until tender. Remove from heat, dissolve miso in 4 tablespoons warm water, and add to pasta. Top with tamari and toasted sesame oil, stir and serve.

Miso-Tahini Spread/Sauce:
Makes approximately ½ to ¾ cup sauce
4 tablespoons tahini (sesame butter)
4 tablespoons water
1 tablespoon traditional barley or red miso
1 tablespoon fresh lemon juice
1 tablespoon minced scallion (optional)

To prepare this quick, versatile sauce, soften miso in water and mix until smooth. Add tahini and lemon juice, again mixing until smooth. Add scallion and serve. Use on grains, vegetables, or on broiled tofu. Add a little more water and you have a delicious salad dressing.

Aihan's Special Foods

Crispy Spring Roll

Serves 4 to 6

Ingredients:
1 pound cabbage, cut into thin strips
1 packet scallion, cut in 1 inch pieces
½ pound chicken, cut into thin strips
5 pieces Chinese dried mushrooms (soaked 30 minutes and boiled)
salt and pepper, to taste
2 teaspoons vegetable or olive oil
1 package spring roll wrap (from Asian grocery stores)
Put two teaspoons of oil in the wok and cook the chicken strips. Put mushroom and cabbage in the wok, add salt and pepper, stir-fry until everything is fully cooked; turn off stove and add scallion. Put them in a bowl. These are fillings for the spring rolls.
Lay out single sheet of roll wrap, put appropriate amount filling in the wrap, roll the wrap by folding a corner first, then folding the side, and finally folding to make a roll.

In the wok, heat the oil, put the rolls in the wok, and deep-fry until golden brown; turn the roll to fry other side. When both sides turn golden brown, pick out the roll from wok and drain the excess oil. Serve with duck sauce and Chinese mustard.

Rice Porridge

Serves 8

This food is popular for sick people and can be used for those who have poor health or poor digestion. It is often used when people catch a cold. The porridge is very light and easy to digest. It is often eaten as a regular breakfast.

Ingredients:
1 cup short rice
5 or 6 cups water, to taste

Put rice and water in a big pot and bring to a boil. Reduce heat to medium and uncover the pot. Cook for 40 minutes. You can add whatever flavor you wish. Most Chinese do not add anything, others add sugar. Try cooking the porridge several ways to find your own favorite combination.

Pork Celery Strings

Serves 2 to 3

Ingredients:
¼ pound pork, cut into 1½ inch long strings
½ pound celery, cut into 1½ inch long strings
1 teaspoon starch, mixed with ¼ cup water
2 tablespoons vegetable oil
¼ teaspoon salt
1 tablespoon soy sauce

Marinate pork with starch and salt for half an hour. Put 2 tablespoons vegetable oil in a hot wok; add pork and stir until mixed well. Once pork is cooked, add celery to the wok and stir for two minutes. Serve with rice.

Students and Patients Speak

Over the years, several of my students and patients have written about their experiences with Chinese medicine and natural healing at my clinic. They are all Westerners who have chosen to explore the 4,000-year-old way to health. Below are a few of those letters that I hope illuminate the power of Traditional Chinese Medicine. As a matter of privacy, I have withheld the names of these patients and students.

In August of 1986, I was diagnosed with mononucleosis, or what we called "the kissing disease," a highly contagious virus that usually affects adolescents. In August of 1987, I was diagnosed with mono again. In August of 1988 I was diagnosed with mono for the third time, and my doctor began a series of blood tests, which proved her diagnosis—Chronic Mono, or what was at that time called Chronic Epstein's Barr Syndrome. Today it is known as Chronic Fatigue Syndrome.

Over the next 15 years, my life was dramatically altered. At the time of my diagnosis, I was Educational Director of a Montessori school. I was also married and we had 3 very active kids, aged 10, 13, and 15, and I taught art to children in our home. At first, I tried to abbreviate my work, but eventually I had to stop working completely.

Two factors helped me to survive all those years of feeling as if I had the flu 24/7.

The first is that I have a wonderful husband who took over more and more of my responsibilities, until he was doing everything, while I napped, ran fevers, and ached. What a pair we made! He worked full-time, did all of the activities with our children, paid all the bills, and did all of the yard work and all of the housework. I napped.

The second helping factor is that in 1994 I learned a meditation practice called surat shabd yoga. Meditation brought peace and happiness into my life—a peace and happiness that all of the doctors and specialists who I saw could not understand. I could not rationally understand it, either. I had every reason to be depressed but I was not. I was happy and peaceful and accepted my illness.

In the summer of 2004, my daughter, who is a nurse at Boston Children's Hospital, went to a conference on Chinese medicine, and the speaker was Dr. Aihan Kuhn. At that time, daughter was wearing leg braces because physical therapy had not worked to relieve the back and knee pain she developed while carrying her first baby. My daughter was so impressed with Dr. Kuhn that she went to her for treatment the following week, and her health improved so quickly that she made an appointment for me to go in early August.

When I went to see Dr. Kuhn for the first time, I was feeling worse than I ever had. I could not stand for 10 seconds without feeling faint; I ate nuts most of the time because they required no preparation. I remember wanting blueberries but I did not have the strength to wash them, and watermelon, but I did not have the strength to cut it. My husband went to concerts and to visit friends alone time after time, because I could not handle the car ride. I could not sit up for a couple of hours straight. I could not hold my head up. I could not sit on most chairs. I could not walk, stand, or sit without pain, and most of the time I had no voice; I was awake at night and asleep during the day. I felt my life was winding down.

That first visit to Dr. Kuhn was a very big deal to me. Although I love my personal doctor who has done all she can to help me, I did not like seeing specialists because it seemed I always felt worse after trying their ideas. My personal doctor told me many times that they just do not know very much about viruses and that was the bottom line.

Because I could not drive to Dr. Kuhn's office, my daughter drove me and I remember barely being able to make it up the flight of stairs. When I went in, Dr. Kuhn came around the desk to meet me. I liked her immediately.

During the first visit, Dr. Kuhn asked me many questions about my health history, and she took my pulse and looked at my tongue. That was it. She made her diagnosis and was ready to begin an acupuncture treatment. Because I lived about 90 miles away, I told Dr. Kuhn I would not be able to come back. She explained to me that with Chinese medicine, a gradual improvement occurs over a period of time and a series of treatments. I told her I would try to come back "some other time," and she gave me two bottles of herbs to take daily at home. She also taped herbs to my ears.

That evening when I got home, I felt wide-awake and was very talkative. Coincidentally, it was our 32nd wedding anniversary, and when my husband asked me if I wanted to eat out or order in, he was very surprised at my wanting to go to a Mexican restaurant. I chatted nonstop to him about Dr. Kuhn. "She's pretty and sweet and I like her office and it didn't hurt to receive the acupuncture," and on and on. Finally, my husband asked me what that lady had given me—speed? We had a good laugh.

Dr. Kuhn had also asked me to do several things daily at home… drink 8 to 10 glasses of water per day, do a series of mild, stretching exercises called Chi Gong, walk half a mile, and take the herbs. I did them all. I decided to try Dr. Kuhn's treatment for a few days, because I felt something was different from just that one visit.

Before a week was up, I called Dr. Kuhn to set up a second appointment. When I went in to see her again, she asked if I could stay at Jena's for a few days and see her twice a week for two weeks. I did. By the time I went back to our home in Connecticut after the two weeks of walking, Chi Gong, herbs, water, and acupuncture, I couldn't talk about anything except how much better I felt. The first week that I was back home again, my best friend, Clare, called to say she would drive me up for my next appointment. While there, she decided to make an appointment for herself and since then we have gone together every week. And, every week I feel better, stronger, and healthier.

That was 12 weeks ago. I now practice Chi Gong daily, take a 2-mile walk 3 or 4 times a week, take my herbs, drink my water, and nap for about 1 hour each day. I sleep at night and am awake during the day. I run up the steps, visit friends and relatives with my husband, and have plans to attend a concert with him in a few weeks. I feel in my heart that I will always need to be careful and keep my life balanced, as Dr. Kuhn teaches, but I also feel in my heart that my life is not unwinding anymore. It feels like I am waking up from a long sleep.

Dr. Kuhn's philosophy is that putting a life back into balance can cure many illnesses. She does her work, the acupuncture treatments, and herbs, and if the patient does his/hers, the Chi Gong and walking, the patient will come into a healthier life. She is smart, compassionate, honest, and very easy to talk to. She knows secrets that the doctors in Western medicine, well intentioned as they are, do not know. I hope the day comes when both East and West join hands in the medical community for the betterment of us all, and if there is anyone who is working hard to bring this about, it is Dr. Kuhn. If you are ill and cannot seem to get better, I highly recommend you visit a woman who has studied both Eastern and Western medicine, and who is performing "little miracles" in Holliston every day.

—B. J. B.

I have been meaning to write to you for sometime. I want to let you know with my sincerest thanks how grateful I am to you for the care you have given me. It is difficult to explain how your treatment has changed my life. I think the best way to say it is to say that you gave me my life back.

When I met you, I was 30 years old and a mother of one, a two-year-old son. I was having pains in my legs that caused me to have difficulty walking (especially on stairs, and especially carrying anything, which is difficult when you are a mom). I also had back pain, which I have had beginning in high school, which when it flared up left me in tears, lying on the floor. I was having trouble working (I am a nurse, and am very physically active at work). My pains were getting worse, and kept me up at night, worrying and in pain. Where would I end up?

I had been to doctors and physical therapy. They meant well but they had no answers and solutions. The best they had was some tight foam braces that cut into my legs and cut off my circulation. I had no choice but to wear them. They kept me walking. I could not believe this was my fate at 30 years old.

I was nervous about trying acupuncture. I did not understand it, and I was not sure it was the right treatment for my pain. You were so caring and reassuring. You let me know right away that there was nothing seriously wrong with me, and how long treatments would take. I decided to go ahead with whatever you said. It was the right choice. You started me on Qigong exercise, which was a key to my healing, which is still a necessary part of my day. And you told me to come twice a week for acupuncture. The treatment was fine, not painless, but not painful. The exercise is not time consuming or difficult.

In just a few months, my pains had completely disappeared. I was able to climb stairs normally, work normally, chase after my son, and even consider having another child. I felt terrific. You even helped me to get pregnant the second time; when, after "trying" for a year, I was still not pregnant, you suggested acupuncture for fertility treatment. You said the treatment usually took three months to work. In three months, I was pregnant.

I am so grateful to have such a kind, understanding, and knowledgeable doctor. I thank God for you and for the work you do. There are others, who practice Chinese medicine, but you are a true healer, and I am so glad I have you for mine.

—J.M.

Thank you for accepting me into your Intensive Care program. I am alive and relatively pain-free, thanks to your care.

I arrived on your doorstep in agony the day after I was told by a neurosurgeon that I would have to have brain surgery (a decompression) to alleviate the pressure of the fluid in my skull. I had undergone brain surgery (shunt) twice before, and was still not convinced it would solve my problem. I was in a lot of pain; could not walk, or even sit for any length of time.

I am a mother of eight and a newspaper photographer and a librarian. I need to walk and sit, and the less pain the better. I have a disease called syringomyelia, which affects the spinal chord, nerves, limbs, brain, and related functions.

Your Intensive Care program included herbal pills, Qigong, and healing massage. We frequently discussed my progress (or lack thereof) and readjusted our "plan of attack." After nine months, the head pain is no longer an issue. I have more energy, less depression, and feel kind of "normal" (I just get ordinary aches and pains). It's so cool.

Thank you so much for all the time and attention, and for giving me an alternative to surgery ("been there—done that—no thanks!").

I hope that I will see you soon for another "tune-up."

—C.M.

I just wanted to write and tell you how great and happy that I have been feeling since I've been coming to you, even though it has only been a few short weeks. I already feel like a new person inside and out. I know the Chi Gong exercises have kept me healthy, too! I have to say this is the first time in years that I have not gotten one cold, and I know it is from doing the Chi Gong exercises. I am so happy and grateful just to know you, Aihan, because I truly feel that you do care about people and want to help them. I also love your bubbly personality and (that you) always look on the positive side of things. I know myself I have always tried to be positive, because the way I see, it, things go better for you when you are positive and your body feels lighter. When you are negative, things do not go as well and your body feels much heavier. It takes fewer muscles to smile than to frown. When you feel good about yourself, you can make the people around you feel good, too. A little smile goes a long way. I know the Chi Gong exercises have made me so far a calmer person, not so nervous. Aihan, I also want to tell you that I think you are a wonderful, kind, caring, and sincere person. I enjoy the Chi Gong classes and plan to take more. I enjoy the meetings. I think I can learn a lot from them and it is nice just to be around such nice people. I know if I keep doing the Chi Gong exercises I can stay healthy and grow old gracefully and happy. Anyway, Aihan, I thank you a thousand times and more for making my life better and keeping me healthy. P.S., I thank Mary Lou for recommending me to you. I love taking the Chi Gong classes with Jean. I think she is great, too!

—F.M.

I am a 72-year old woman who has been a participant in Oriental exercise classes taught by Aihan Kuhn once weekly for approximately a year and have found them to be good for my physical and mental well-being.

Since the exercises are enjoyable as well as beneficial, I do them on my own at home between classes. I consider the time to be very well spent. The benefits are achieved without the necessity of quick, jerky movements and over-strenuous activity. There is no possibility for injury because of the teacher's caring and attention to each student's needs.

Specific benefits that I have experienced are increased vitality and flexibility resulting in fewer aches and pains that are a part of the aging process. It is wonderful to have a back or headache seldom. Very importantly, stress reduction for me has occurred naturally, creating physical and mental harmony.

It is with great confidence I can recommend Oriental Exercise classes for all ages, and especially for the elderly.

—N.H.

May I take this opportunity to let you know how much I enjoy the oriental class that you teach? At the end of the exercise class, my mind and body feel so relaxed. I concentrate solely on what I am doing. The exercise helps all parts of my body—from the top of my head to my feet. And I must tell you it also helps to keep my blood pressure down.

I look forward to your class every week. Keep up the good work. It keeps our bodies in shape and alleviates some of our body pains.

—G.J.

When I first came to see Dr. Aihan Kuhn, I was very sick. I had been sick for two years. Recovering from a hysterectomy, I had many complications, anxiety, depression, urinary tract infections, and yeast and bacteria infections. Eight months before that, I had a breast biopsy. Headaches and fatigue were horrible. I felt terrible from constant panic attacks. I didn't know what else to do, and my doctors were getting nowhere with me, but giving me more antibiotics, which made me worse.

Dr. Aihan Kuhn explained Chinese medicine to me. I was very skeptical and frightened. I recall her words "don't worry," "don't worry," she said. That day, she did acupressure on my ear and immediately I felt better. She sent me home with tea to make and drink for a week. After that week, I felt better.

Weeks later, she did acupuncture on my bladder and I am doing quite well. I have also had acupuncture on my back for arthritis and the pain and swelling are almost gone. It has now been nine months and I think my progress has been very good. I have also learned Taiji and Chi Gong. These classes are a lot of hard work because you must practice a lot but it is a lot of fun and very rewarding.

I never dreamed I could learn Taiji, but everyone in the classes I took were so helpful and gave me so much encouragement. My first class was so stressful because I was so scared. My hands and knees were shaking so hard I remember saying to myself, "I am so nervous, how can I even learn this, this is impossible." Everyone in the class said to me "don't stop trying, you'll get it, it takes time and practice." Okay I said and I practiced every day, every week for weeks and finally one week I got it. It just clicked in and I did it. I did Taiji! I was so proud of myself and so thankful for meeting such wonderful people who helped me and gave me all this encouragement.

Now I do Taiji and Chi Gong morning and night. It keeps me in balance and very healthy. I have more energy and less pain and disease. Dr. Aihan Kuhn is a remarkable person. I listen to everything she tells me and teaches me. She takes the time to talk to you no matter how busy she is. She cares about people, she is very honest and strict. She expects nothing but the best you can do and she always has your best interest in mind. I respect her so much as a person, teacher, philosopher, and Doctor of Medicine. Alternative medicine, Dr. Aihan Kuhn, and many people in her classes have helped me tremendously in my healing. I thank everyone from the bottom of my heart.

—M.W.

I am 84 years old and Chi Gong is part of my life.

I tell everyone about it and most people do not know what it is. For many years, I have watched the people of China do their exercises out in the parks and many of them are old people. I think of myself and how good I feel. Some mornings I do not feel too well and I feel like skipping them but I talk myself out of feeling sorry for myself and I put in the tape. The music calms me and I get to work. I have not mastered the deep breathing yet. I know that when you breathe deeply your brain gets more oxygen and that helps you think more clearly.

I think that if you do your exercises in the open air like on the town common people will take notice and become interested. People are curious and when they hear the music they will stop and see what is going on.

We in America are all out of shape. Most workers just sit at a desk all day. I myself, when I worked as a welder for General Electric, just sat at my machine all day. The only exercise I got was working with my hands.

I think industry should lay aside some time for a little workout to change the positions and breathe new life into our robotic souls.

Chi Gong could be taught in schools in the Gym class. When I think of it I looked forward to Gym and I always got an A. One of the very few that I got.

Now I am busy nearly every day and I tell my friends that I keep moving so the Grim Reaper will not know where I am.

These are my thoughts that are written here, they may not be of any value but just a few words to let you know how I feel and to thank you for giving me the privilege to strengthen my body.

—L.D.

Further Readings

Historical References
Huang Di Nei Jing (*Yellow Emperor's Classic of Internal Medicine*)
Golden Principle—A Guide for Medical Workers
Lei Jing Tu Yi (*The Illustrated Supplement to the Categorized Canon*)
Materia Medica (*Ben Chao Gang Mu*)

Books

Beinfield, Harriet and Korngold, Efrem. 1992. *Between Heaven and Earth. A Guide to Chinese Medicine*. New York: Ballantine Wellspring (Random House, Inc.). Clear explanations to help the beginner understand Chinese medicine.

Dalton, Jerry O. 1996. *Tao Te Ching: A New Approach*. Backward Down the Path. New York: Avon Books.

Douglas, Bill. 1998. *The Complete Idiot's Guide to T'ai Chi and Qigong*. New York, NY: Alpha Books. An excellent book for beginners who have never been exposed to Taiji and Qigong.

Hadady, Letha. 1996. *Asian Health Secrets: The Complete Guide to Asian Herbal Medicine*. New York: Crown Publishers

Huang, Li-Chen, *Auriculotherapy: Diagnoses and Treatment*. (trans. Quan Zhou and Elaine Murphy). Bellaire, TX: Longevity Press.

Kuhn, Aihan. 2003. *Tai Chi Student Handbook. Chinese Medicine for Health*. Holliston, MA: New England School of Tai Chi.

Kuhn, Aihan. 2004. *Natural Healing with Qigong. Therapeutic Qigong*. Boston, MA: YMAA Publication Center.

Kuhn, Aihan. 2006. *Tai Chi for Depression*. Holliston, MA: New England School of Tai Chi.

Kushi, Michio and Stephen Blauer. 2004. *The Macrobiotic Way: The Complete Macrobiotic Lifestyle Book*. 3rd Edition. Wayne, NJ: Avery Publishing Group.

Lu, Henry C. 1986. *Chinese System of Food Cures: Prevention &Remedies*. New York: Sterling Publishers Co.

Pitchford, Paul. 2002. *Healing with Whole Foods: Asian Traditions and Modern Nutrition*. Berkeley, CA: North Atlantic Books.

Reid, Daniel. 1994. *The Complete Book of Chinese Health and Healing. Guarding the Three Treasures*. Boston, MA: Shambhala. Helpful for Westerners trying to understand the Chinese style of healing.

Yang, Jwing-Ming. 1997. *Eight Simple Qigong Exercises for Health. The Eight Pieces of Brocade*. 2nd Edition. Boston, MA: YMAA Publication Center.

Yang, Jwing-Ming. 1997. *The Root of Chinese Qigong*. Boston, MA: YMAA Publication Center. For people who really want to explore the true nature of Qigong.

Periodicals
Qi Journal
Empty Vessel

Interesting Internet Sites
See www.religioustolerance.org/Daoism.htm for information about the impact of Daoism in North America.

A comprehensive chart of food's fiber content can be found in http://www.slrhc.org/healthinfo/dietaryfiber/fibercontentchart.html#fiber#fiber.

A list of DVDs and books that my clinic sells can be found at www.taichihealing.com

Index

About the Author

Dr. Aihan Kuhn is a 1982 graduate of Hunan Medical University in China. She has had training in both conventional Western and Traditional Chinese Medicine. For six years, prior to coming to United States in 1989, she practiced in a hospital in China as an OB-GYN doctor. In her practice she was able to use both Western and Chinese medicine. Since she was 10 years old she has been interested in Chinese Martial Arts, and has studied sword exercise. She has always been interested in nature, and natural cures for sickness. In 1978, she started to study Qigong, Taiji, and other oriental exercises. She started to teach in China in 1984 and has been teaching in the United States since 1992.

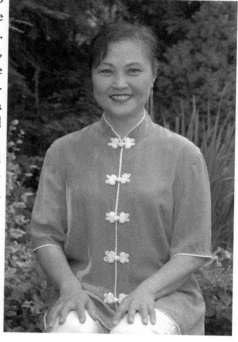

Dr. Kuhn believes that maintaining good health and preventing illness is more important than treating disease. To achieve a healthy lifestyle, Dr. Kuhn has found that one should work hard on improving Qi (the life force that is within us.) She focuses on healthy ways of thinking and eating, routine Chinese exercise to enhance energy flow, and the practice of Traditional Chinese Medicine to help others to get well. To share her knowledge and experience in ancient Chinese healing, Dr. Kuhn has provided many on-site workshops and seminars to hospital professionals, wellness centers, senior centers, schools and colleges, nursing homes, and companies. Periodic lectures, as well as Continuing Education Unit (CEU) programs for Nurses and Physical Therapists, are held in her clinic. Dr. Kuhn has been teaching Taiji, Qigong and other healing exercises in the United States since 1992. She is a unique "Natural Psychologist" who searches for wisdom from nature. She has a reputation as being "the best teacher and instructor," "an excellent speaker and lecturer," "a wonderful healer," and "an amazing doctor, [which is very] hard to find."

Dr. Kuhn is a Massachusetts State sponsor for World Taiji and Qigong Day, an international event created to promote and foster awareness of the health benefits of practicing Taiji and Qigong. Taiji and Qigong groups all over the world go out and practice in public parks on this same day and hour to spread the healing spirit.

Dr. Kuhn is the director and owner of Chinese Medicine for Health, New England School of Taiji. She is President and founder of the Taiji and Qigong Healing

Institute (TQHI.) This is a non-profit organization focused on education and the study of human natural energy science and its healing effects in order to provide access to an improved quality of life. TQHI is committed to improving health care using traditional Chinese healing arts such as Qigong and Taiji, to improve body energy circulation in order to maintain optimum health and heal ailments, including some for which Western medicine has no cure.

Dr. Aihan Kuhn, C.M.D., DIPL. ABT.
Master, Tai Chi and Qi Gong
Chinese Medicine for Health, Inc.
New England School of Tai Chi
1564A Washington Street
Holliston, MA 01746
(508) 429-3895
35 Kingston Street
Boston, MA
(617 981-2039)

www.chinesemedicineforhealth.com
drkuhn@chinesemedicineforhealth.com

101 REFLECTIONS ON TAI CHI CHUAN
108 INSIGHTS INTO TAI CHI CHUAN
A SUDDEN DAWN: THE EPIC JOURNEY OF BODHIDHARMA
A WOMAN'S QIGONG GUIDE
ADVANCING IN TAE KWON DO
ANALYSIS OF SHAOLIN CHIN NA 2ND ED
ANCIENT CHINESE WEAPONS
THE ART AND SCIENCE OF STAFF FIGHTING
THE ART AND SCIENCE OF STICK FIGHTING
ART OF HOJO UNDO
ARTHRITIS RELIEF, 3D ED.
BACK PAIN RELIEF, 2ND ED.
BAGUAZHANG, 2ND ED.
BRAIN FITNESS
CARDIO KICKBOXING ELITE
CHIN NA IN GROUND FIGHTING
CHINESE FAST WRESTLING
CHINESE FITNESS
CHINESE TUI NA MASSAGE
CHOJUN
COMPLETE MARTIAL ARTIST
COMPREHENSIVE APPLICATIONS OF SHAOLIN CHIN NA
CONFLICT COMMUNICATION
CROCODILE AND THE CRANE: A NOVEL
CUTTING SEASON: A XENON PEARL MARTIAL ARTS THRILLER
DAO DE JING
DAO IN ACTION
DEFENSIVE TACTICS
DESHI: A CONNOR BURKE MARTIAL ARTS THRILLER
DIRTY GROUND
DR. WU'S HEAD MASSAGE
DUKKHA HUNGRY GHOSTS
DUKKHA REVERB
DUKKHA, THE SUFFERING: AN EYE FOR AN EYE
DUKKHA UNLOADED
ENZAN: THE FAR MOUNTAIN, A CONNOR BURKE MARTIAL ARTS
    THRILLER
ESSENCE OF SHAOLIN WHITE CRANE
EVEN IF IT KILLS ME
EXPLORING TAI CHI
FACING VIOLENCE
FIGHT BACK
FIGHT LIKE A PHYSICIST
THE FIGHTER'S BODY
FIGHTER'S FACT BOOK
FIGHTER'S FACT BOOK 2
THE FIGHTING ARTS
FIGHTING THE PAIN RESISTANT ATTACKER
FIRST DEFENSE
FORCE DECISIONS: A CITIZENS GUIDE
FOX BORROWS THE TIGER'S AWE
INSIDE TAI CHI
THE JUDO ADVANTAGE
THE JUJI GATAME ENCYCLOPEDIA
KAGE: THE SHADOW, A CONNOR BURKE MARTIAL ARTS THRILLER
KARATE SCIENCE
KATA AND THE TRANSMISSION OF KNOWLEDGE
KRAV MAGA COMBATIVES
KRAV MAGA PROFESSIONAL TACTICS
KRAV MAGA WEAPON DEFENSES
LITTLE BLACK BOOK OF VIOLENCE
LIUHEBAFA FIVE CHARACTER SECRETS
MARTIAL ARTS ATHLETE
MARTIAL ARTS INSTRUCTION
MARTIAL WAY AND ITS VIRTUES
MASK OF THE KING
MEDITATIONS ON VIOLENCE
MERIDIAN QIGONG EXERCISES
MIND/BODY FITNESS
MINDFUL EXERCISE
THE MIND INSIDE TAI CHI
THE MIND INSIDE YANG STYLE TAI CHI CHUAN
MUGAI RYU
NATURAL HEALING WITH QIGONG
NORTHERN SHAOLIN SWORD, 2ND ED.
OKINAWA'S COMPLETE KARATE SYSTEM: ISSHIN RYU
THE PAIN-FREE BACK

PAIN-FREE JOINTS
POWER BODY
PRINCIPLES OF TRADITIONAL CHINESE MEDICINE
THE PROTECTOR ETHIC
QIGONG FOR HEALTH & MARTIAL ARTS 2ND ED.
QIGONG FOR LIVING
QIGONG FOR TREATING COMMON AILMENTS
QIGONG MASSAGE
QIGONG MEDITATION: EMBRYONIC BREATHING
QIGONG MEDITATION: SMALL CIRCULATION
QIGONG, THE SECRET OF YOUTH: DA MO'S CLASSICS
QUIET TEACHER: A XENON PEARL MARTIAL ARTS THRILLER
RAVEN'S WARRIOR
REDEMPTION
ROOT OF CHINESE QIGONG, 2ND ED.
SAMBO ENCYCLOPEDIA
SCALING FORCE
SELF-DEFENSE FOR WOMEN
SENSEI: A CONNOR BURKE MARTIAL ARTS THRILLER
SHIHAN TE: THE BUNKAI OF KATA
SHIN GI TAI: KARATE TRAINING FOR BODY, MIND, AND SPIRIT
SIMPLE CHINESE MEDICINE
SIMPLE QIGONG EXERCISES FOR HEALTH, 3RD ED.
SIMPLIFIED TAI CHI CHUAN, 2ND ED.
SOLO TRAINING
SOLO TRAINING 2
SPOTTING DANGER BEFORE DANGER SPOTS YOU
SUMO FOR MIXED MARTIAL ARTS
SUNRISE TAI CHI
SUNSET TAI CHI
SURVIVING ARMED ASSAULTS
TAE KWON DO: THE KOREAN MARTIAL ART
TAEKWONDO BLACK BELT POOMSAE
TAEKWONDO: A PATH TO EXCELLENCE
TAEKWONDO: ANCIENT WISDOM FOR THE MODERN WARRIOR
TAEKWONDO: DEFENSE AGAINST WEAPONS
TAEKWONDO: SPIRIT AND PRACTICE
TAO OF BIOENERGETICS
TAI CHI BALL QIGONG: FOR HEALTH AND MARTIAL ARTS
TAI CHI BALL WORKOUT FOR BEGINNERS
THE TAI CHI BOOK
TAI CHI CHIN NA: THE SEIZING ART OF TAI CHI CHUAN,
    2ND ED.
TAI CHI CHUAN CLASSICAL YANG STYLE, 2ND ED.
TAI CHI CHUAN MARTIAL POWER, 3RD ED.
TAI CHI CONNECTIONS
TAI CHI DYNAMICS
TAI CHI FOR DEPRESSION
TAI CHI IN 10 WEEKS
TAI CHI QIGONG, 3RD ED.
TAI CHI SECRETS OF THE ANCIENT MASTERS
TAI CHI SECRETS OF THE WU & LI STYLES
TAI CHI SECRETS OF THE WU STYLE
TAI CHI SECRETS OF THE YANG STYLE
TAI CHI SWORD: CLASSICAL YANG STYLE, 2ND ED.
TAI CHI SWORD FOR BEGINNERS
TAI CHI WALKING
TAIJIQUAN THEORY OF DR. YANG, JWING-MING
TAO OF BIOENERGETICS
TENGU: THE MOUNTAIN GOBLIN, A CONNOR BURKE MARTIAL ARTS
    THRILLER
TIMING IN THE FIGHTING ARTS
TRADITIONAL CHINESE HEALTH SECRETS
TRADITIONAL TAEKWONDO
TRAINING FOR SUDDEN VIOLENCE
TRUE WELLNESS
TRUE WELLNESS: THE MIND
TRUE WELLNESS: THE HEART
THE WARRIOR'S MANIFESTO
WAY OF KATA
WAY OF KENDO AND KENJITSU
WAY OF SANCHIN KATA
WAY TO BLACK BELT
WESTERN HERBS FOR MARTIAL ARTISTS
WILD GOOSE QIGONG
WINNING FIGHTS
WISDOM'S WAY
XINGYIQUAN

DVDS FROM YMAA

ADVANCED PRACTICAL CHIN NA IN-DEPTH
ANALYSIS OF SHAOLIN CHIN NA
ATTACK THE ATTACK
BAGUA FOR BEGINNERS 1
BAGUA FOR BEGINNERS 2
BAGUAZHANG: EMEI BAGUAZHANG
BEGINNER QIGONG FOR WOMEN 1
BEGINNER QIGONG FOR WOMEN 2
BEGINNER TAI CHI FOR HEALTH
CHEN STYLE TAIJIQUAN
CHEN TAI CHI FOR BEGINNERS
CHIN NA IN-DEPTH COURSES 1—4
CHIN NA IN-DEPTH COURSES 5—8
CHIN NA IN-DEPTH COURSES 9—12
FACING VIOLENCE: 7 THINGS A MARTIAL ARTIST MUST KNOW
FIVE ANIMAL SPORTS
FIVE ELEMENTS ENERGY BALANCE
INFIGHTING
INTRODUCTION TO QI GONG FOR BEGINNERS
JOINT LOCKS
KNIFE DEFENSE: TRADITIONAL TECHNIQUES AGAINST A DAGGER
KUNG FU BODY CONDITIONING 1
KUNG FU BODY CONDITIONING 2
KUNG FU FOR KIDS
KUNG FU FOR TEENS
LOGIC OF VIOLENCE
MERIDIAN QIGONG
NEIGONG FOR MARTIAL ARTS
NORTHERN SHAOLIN SWORD : SAN CAI JIAN, KUN WU JIAN, QI MEN JIAN
QI GONG 30-DAY CHALLENGE
QI GONG FOR ANXIETY
QI GONG FOR ARMS, WRISTS, AND HANDS
QIGONG FOR BEGINNERS: FRAGRANCE
QI GONG FOR BETTER BREATHING
QI GONG FOR CANCER
QI GONG FOR ENERGY AND VITALITY
QI GONG FOR HEADACHES
QI GONG FOR HEALING
QI GONG FOR HEALTHY JOINTS
QI GONG FOR HIGH BLOOD PRESSURE
QIGONG FOR LONGEVITY
QI GONG FOR STRONG BONES
QI GONG FOR THE UPPER BACK AND NECK
QIGONG FOR WOMEN
QIGONG FOR WOMEN WITH DAISY LEE
QIGONG MASSAGE
QIGONG MINDFULNESS IN MOTION
QIGONG: 15 MINUTES TO HEALTH
SABER FUNDAMENTAL TRAINING
SAI TRAINING AND SEQUENCES
SANCHIN KATA: TRADITIONAL TRAINING FOR KARATE POWER
SCALING FORCE
SHAOLIN KUNG FU FUNDAMENTAL TRAINING: COURSES 1 & 2
SHAOLIN LONG FIST KUNG FU: ADVANCED SEQUENCES 1
SHAOLIN LONG FIST KUNG FU: ADVANCED SEQUENCES 2
SHAOLIN LONG FIST KUNG FU: BASIC SEQUENCES
SHAOLIN LONG FIST KUNG FU: INTERMEDIATE SEQUENCES
SHAOLIN SABER: BASIC SEQUENCES
SHAOLIN STAFF: BASIC SEQUENCES
SHAOLIN WHITE CRANE GONG FU BASIC TRAINING: COURSES 1 & 2

SHAOLIN WHITE CRANE GONG FU BASIC TRAINING: COURSES 3 & 4
SHUAI JIAO: KUNG FU WRESTLING
SIMPLE QIGONG EXERCISES FOR HEALTH
SIMPLE QIGONG EXERCISES FOR ARTHRITIS RELIEF
SIMPLE QIGONG EXERCISES FOR BACK PAIN RELIEF
SIMPLIFIED TAI CHI CHUAN: 24 & 48 POSTURES
SIMPLIFIED TAI CHI FOR BEGINNERS 48
SUNRISE TAI CHI
SUNSET TAI CHI
SWORD: FUNDAMENTAL TRAINING
TAEKWONDO KORYO POOMSAE
TAI CHI BALL QIGONG: COURSES 1 & 2
TAI CHI BALL QIGONG: COURSES 3 & 4
TAI CHI BALL WORKOUT FOR BEGINNERS
TAI CHI CHUAN CLASSICAL YANG STYLE
TAI CHI CONNECTIONS
TAI CHI ENERGY PATTERNS
TAI CHI FIGHTING SET
TAI CHI FIT: 24 FORM
TAI CHI FIT: FLOW
TAI CHI FIT: FUSION BAMBOO
TAI CHI FIT: FUSION FIRE
TAI CHI FIT: FUSION IRON
TAI CHI FIT IN PARADISE
TAI CHI FIT: OVER 50
TAI CHI FIT OVER 50: SEATED WORKOUT FOR HEALTH
TAI CHI FIT OVER 50: BALANCE EXERCISES
TAI CHI FIT OVER 60: HEALTHY JOINTS
TAI CHI FIT OVER 60: LIVE LONGER, FEEL YOUNGER
TAI CHI FIT: STRENGTH
TAI CHI FIT: TO GO
TAI CHI FOR WOMEN
TAI CHI FUSION: FIRE
TAI CHI QIGONG
TAI CHI PUSHING HANDS: COURSES 1 & 2
TAI CHI PUSHING HANDS: COURSES 3 & 4
TAI CHI SWORD: CLASSICAL YANG STYLE
TAI CHI SWORD FOR BEGINNERS
TAI CHI SYMBOL: YIN YANG STICKING HANDS
TAIJI & SHAOLIN STAFF: FUNDAMENTAL TRAINING
TAIJI CHIN NA IN-DEPTH
TAIJI 37 POSTURES MARTIAL APPLICATIONS
TAIJI SABER CLASSICAL YANG STYLE
TAIJI WRESTLING
TRAINING FOR SUDDEN VIOLENCE
UNDERSTANDING QIGONG 1: WHAT IS QI? • HUMAN QI
  CIRCULATORY SYSTEM
UNDERSTANDING QIGONG 2: KEY POINTS • QIGONG BREATHING
UNDERSTANDING QIGONG 3: EMBRYONIC BREATHING
UNDERSTANDING QIGONG 4: FOUR SEASONS QIGONG
UNDERSTANDING QIGONG 5: SMALL CIRCULATION
UNDERSTANDING QIGONG 6: MARTIAL QIGONG BREATHING
WATER STYLE FOR BEGINNERS
WHITE CRANE HARD & SOFT QIGONG
YANG TAI CHI FOR BEGINNERSS
WUDANG KUNG FU: FUNDAMENTAL TRAINING
WUDANG SWORD
WUDANG TAIJIQUAN
XINGYIQUAN
YANG TAI CHI FOR BEGINNERS

more products available from . . .

YMAA Publication Center, Inc. 楊氏東方文化出版中心

1-800-669-8892 • info@ymaa.com • www.ymaa.com